Keto Diet Cookbook

The best beginner's guide over 250 recipes Quick and Easy to Heal
Your Body and Lose Your Weight

James Lewis

Table of Contents

Introduction

Under the ketogenic diet, the body is pushed to the state of ketosis wherein it uses up fat bodies called ketones as its main source of energy instead of glucose. Unlike other short-lived fad diets, the ketogenic diet has been around for more than ninety years as it was first used to treat patients who suffered from epilepsy. Today, it is still used to minimize the effects of epileptic seizures, but it is also used for weight loss. People who follow the ketogenic diet limit the intake of carbohydrates to around 20 to 30 net grams daily or 5% of the daily diet. Net grams refer to the number of carbohydrates that remain after subtracting the grams of dietary fiber. Since the carbohydrate intake is limited, dieters are encouraged to consume more fat and protein in amounts of 80% and 20%; respectively. The ketogenic diet is often referred to as a low-carb diet, but it is important to take note that it [ketogenic diet] is entirely different from the other low-carb diets that encourage protein loading. Protein is not as important as fat is in the ketogenic diet. The reason is that the presence of a higher amount of protein pushes the body to the process called gluconeogenesis wherein protein is converted into glucose. If this happens, the body is not pushed to a state of ketosis. This is the reason why it is so crucial to consume more fat under the ketogenic diet than protein. When we eat, the carbohydrates found in the food that we consume is converted into a simple sugar called glucose. Alongside converting carbs to glucose, the pancreas also manufactures insulin, which is a hormone responsible for pushing glucose into the cells to be used up as energy. Keto Diet Cookbook As glucose is used up as the main source of energy, the fats that you also consume from food is not utilized thus they are immediately stored in the liver and adipocytes (specialized fat cells). Moreover, if you consume too many carbohydrates, the glucose that is not used up is converted into glycogen and is stored in the liver and muscles as standby energy source. If not used up, it is processed and converted to fat and stored all over the body, thus you gain weight. However, the body is working in a brilliant system that allows us to use up and burn off fats from our body. The ability of the body to produce ketones is part of the millions of years of the human evolution. It protected our ancestors during times of starvation in the past. During periods of famines in the past wherein the body cannot consume carbohydrates over long periods of time, the body uses up fats as a source of energy, as it does in ketosis. This process has helped our ancestors survived for millions of years. Amazing, right? So, when does ketosis happen? People usually enter the state of ketosis after 3 to 4 days consuming little amounts of carbohydrates. But to undergo the state of ketosis, some people think that you must stop eating altogether—but not with the ketogenic diet. The ketogenic diet bypasses starvation by encouraging you to eat more fats and adequate amounts of protein so that you don't have to undergo starvation. So, what food should you eat? This diet regimen encourages people to consume more fats sourced from healthy and whole food ingredients. That way, the body is pushed to a pure state of ketosis without ever feeling hungry.

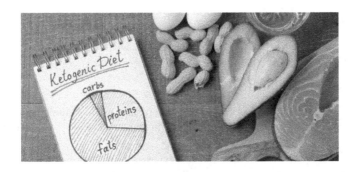

PORK, BEEF & LAMB RECIPES

1. Mom's Meatballs in Creamy Sauce

(Ready in about 30 minutes | Servings 6) Per serving: 378 Calories; 29.9g Fat; 2.9g Carbs; 23.4g Protein; 0.3g

Ingredients For the Meatballs: 2 eggs 1 tablespoon steak seasoning 1 tablespoon green garlic, minced 1 tablespoon scallions, minced 1 pound ground pork 1/2 pound ground turkey For the Sauce: 3 teaspoons ghee 1 cup double cream 1 cup cream of onion soup Salt and pepper, to your liking 1/2 teaspoon dried rosemary

Directions

Preheat your oven to 365 degrees F. In a mixing bowl, combine all ingredients for the meatballs. Roll the mixture into 20 to 24 balls and place them on a parchment-lined baking sheet. Roast for about 25 minutes or until your meatballs are golden-brown on the top. While your meatballs are roasting, melt the ghee in a preheated sauté pan over a moderate flame. Gradually add in the remaining ingredients, whisking constantly, until the sauce has reduced slightly. Bon appétit!

2. Easy Pork Tenderloin Gumbo

(Ready in about 35 minutes | Servings 6) Per serving: 427 Calories; 16.2g Fat; 3.6g Carbs; 33.2g Protein; 4.4g

Ingredients 1 pound pork tenderloin, cubed 8 ounces New Orleans spicy sausage, sliced 1 tablespoon Cajun spice mix 1 medium-sized leek, chopped 2 tablespoons olive oil 5 cups bone broth 1/2 cup celery, chopped 1 teaspoon gumbo file 1/4 cup flaxseed meal 3/4 pound okra 2 bell peppers, deveined and thinly sliced

Directions In a heavy-bottomed pot, heat the oil until sizzling. Sear the pork tenderloin and New Orleans sausage for about 8 minutes or until browned on all sides; set aside. In the same pot, cook the leek and peppers until they softened. Add in the gumbo file, Cajun spice and broth. Bring it to a rolling boil. Turn the heat to medium-low and add in celery. Let it simmer for 18 to 20 minutes longer. Stir in the flax seed meal and okra along with the reserved meat. Then, continue to simmer for 5 to 6 minutes or until heated through. Enjoy!

3. Bacon Blue Cheese Fat Bombs

(Ready in about 5 minutes | Servings 4) Per serving: 232 Calories; 17.6g Fat; 2.9g Carbs; 14.2g Protein; 0.6g

Ingredients

1 ½ tablespoons mayonnaise 1/2 cup bacon, chopped 3 ounces blue cheese, crumbled 3 ounces cream cheese 2 tablespoons chives, chopped 2 teaspoons tomato puree

Directions

Mix all ingredients until everything is well combined. Shape the mixture into 8 equal fat bombs. Serve well chilled!

---

4. German Pork Rouladen

(Ready in about 1 hour + marinating time | Servings 6) Per serving: 220 Calories; 6g Fat; 2.8g Carbs; 33.3g Protein; 0.4g

Ingredients

1 ½ pounds boneless pork loin, butterflied 2 garlic cloves, pressed 1 tablespoon ghee, room temperature 1 tablespoon Mediterranean herb mix 1 teaspoon mustard seeds 1/2 teaspoon cumin seeds 1 cup roasted vegetable broth 1 large-sized onion, thinly sliced Salt and black peppercorns, to taste 1/2 cup Burgundy wine

Directions

Boil the pork loin for about 5 minutes; pat it dry. Now, combine the Mediterranean herb mix, mustard seeds, cumin seeds, garlic and ghee. Unfold the pork loin and spread the rub all over the cut side. Roll the pork and secure with kitchen string. Allow it to sit at least 2 hours in your refrigerator. Place the pork loin in a lightly greased baking pan. Add on wine, broth, onion, salt, and black peppercorns. Roast in the preheated oven at 390 degrees F approximately 1 hour. Bon appétit!

5. Pork and Vegetable Souvlaki

(Ready in about 20 minutes + marinating time | Servings 6) Per serving: 267 Calories; 10.6g Fat; 5.3g Carbs; 34.9g Protein; 1.3g

Ingredients 1 tablespoon Greek spice mix 2 cloves garlic, crushed 3 tablespoons coconut aminos 3 tablespoons olive oil 1 tablespoon stone-ground mustard 2 tablespoons fresh lemon juice 1 pound brown mushrooms 2 bell peppers, cut into thick slices 1 red bell pepper, cut into thick slices 1 zucchini, cubed 1 shallot, cut into wedges 2 pounds pork butt, cubed Bamboo skewers, soaked in cold water for 30 minutes

Directions Mix the Greek spice mix, garlic, coconut aminos, olive oil, mustard, and lemon juice in a ceramic dish; add in pork cubes and let it marinate for 2 hours. Thread the pork cubes and vegetables onto the soaked skewers. Salt to taste. Grill for about 15 minutes, basting with the reserved marinade. Bon appétit!

6. Pork and Broccoli Stew

(Ready in about 2 hours | Servings 6) Per serving: 326 Calories; 13.9g Fat; 6g Carbs; 23.5g Protein; 1.2g

Ingredients

2 tablespoons lard, at room temperature 1 ½ pounds pork shoulder, cubed 1 teaspoon smoked paprika Sea salt and ground black pepper to taste 1 brown onion, chopped 1 stalk celery, chopped 1 teaspoon garlic, finely minced 1/4 cup dry red wine 3 cups water 2 bay leaves 1/2 teaspoon celery seeds 2 bell peppers, chopped 1 chili pepper, chopped 1 cup broccoli, broken into florets 1 tablespoon beef bouillon granules 1 tablespoon flax seed meal

Directions

Melt the lard in a heavy-bottomed pot over a moderate flame. Now, cook the pork for 5 to 6 minutes or until browned on all sides. Season with paprika, salt, and black pepper; reserve. In the same pot, sauté the onion, celery and garlic until they've softened. Add a splash of dry red wine to scrape up any browned bits from the bottom of your pot. Add in the water, bay leaves, celery seeds, bell peppers, and chili pepper. Reduce the temperature to simmer and add in the reserved pork. Continue to simmer for 1 hour 20 minutes. Add in the broccoli and beef bouillon granules and cook an additional 15 minutes. Add in the flax seed meal to thicken the cooking liquid. Taste and adjust the seasonings. Bon appétit!

7. Italian Pork Soup

(Ready in about 1 hour | Servings 4) Per serving: 331 Calories; 17.6g Fat; 4.4g Carbs; 37.4g Protein; 0.9g

Ingredients

1 shallot, chopped 4 cups beef bone broth 1 tomato, crushed 1 Pepperoncini, seeded and cut into very thin strips with scissors 1 tablespoon Italian herb mix 1 teaspoon green garlic, minced 1/2 cup Marsala wine 1 carrot, thinly sliced 2 tablespoons olive oil 1 ½ pounds pork stew meat, cubed 1 Italian pepper, thinly sliced Salt and black pepper, to taste

Directions

In a soup pot, heat the oil over a moderately high flame. Brown the pork for about 6 minutes until no longer pink; set aside. In the same pot, cook the shallot until tender and fragrant. Stir in the garlic and continue to sauté for 30 seconds more or until aromatic. Add in wine to deglaze the bottom of the soup pot. Add in the remaining ingredients along with the reserved pork; bring to a rapid boil. Reduce the heat to medium-low; continue to simmer, partially covered, for about 45 minutes. Bon appétit!

8. Barbecue Saucy Pork

(Ready in about 2 hours | Servings 8) Per serving: 561 Calories; 34g Fat; 1.7g Carbs; 52.7g Protein; 0.4g

Ingredients

2 tablespoons olive oil 1 teaspoon fresh garlic, halved 2 pounds pork butt Sea salt and freshly ground black pepper, to taste 1/3 teaspoon hot paprika A few drops of liquid smoke 1/3 teaspoon ground cumin 1/2 cup marinara sauce 1 teaspoon hot sauce 1 teaspoon stone-ground mustard

Directions

Rub the pork with the olive oil and garlic. Sprinkle with salt, pepper, and hot paprika. Roast the pork at 410 degrees F for 20 minutes. Turn the heat to 340 degrees F and roast for about 1 hour. In a mixing bowl, whisk the remaining ingredients. Spoon the sauce over the pork and continue to roast an additional 20 minutes. Enjoy!

9. Polish Sausage and Sauerkraut

(Ready in about 35 minutes | Servings 6) Per serving: 309 Calories; 20.6g Fat; 4.2g Carbs; 19.3g Protein; 3.8g

Ingredients

4 slices Polish bacon, chopped 2 pork sausages, sliced 1 onion, chopped 1/3 cup dry white wine 1 Serano pepper, finely minced 1 teaspoon garlic, finely minced 1/2 teaspoon fennel seeds, ground 1/2 teaspoon mustard seeds 1 cup vegetable broth 1 ½ pounds prepared sauerkraut, drained

Directions In a saucepan, fry the bacon over medium-high heat for 7 to 8 minutes; reserve. In the same pan, cook the sausage until no longer pink for 4 to 5 minutes; reserve. Then, cook the onions until tender and translucent for 5 to 6 minutes. Add a splash of wine to deglaze the pan. Add in the remaining ingredients and bring to a boil; turn the heat to simmer and continue to cook for 15 to 18 minutes or until everything is cooked through.Bon appétit!

10. Breakfast Mug Muffin

(Ready in about 10 minutes | Servings 2) Per serving: 327 Calories; 16.6g Fat; 5.8g Carbs; 40g Protein; 1.2g

Ingredients 1/2 cup marinara sauce 1/2 cup cheddar cheese, shredded 1/2 pound ground pork 1 teaspoon garlic paste 1/2 teaspoon shallot powder Salt and ground black pepper, to taste 1/2 teaspoon paprika

DirectionsIn a mixing bowl, combine all ingredients until everything is well incorporated. Spoon the mixture into two microwave-safe mugs. Microwave for 5 minutes until set but still moist.Bon appétit!

11. Baked Pork Meatballs in Pasta Sauce

Ready in about: 45 minutes | Serves: 6 Per serving: Kcal 590, Fat 46.8g, Net Carbs 4.1g, Protein 46.2g

Ingredients

2 lb ground pork 1 tbsp olive oil 1 cup pork rinds, crushed 2 cloves garlic, minced ½ cup coconut milk 2 eggs, beaten ½ cup Parmesan cheese, grated ½ cup asiago cheese, grated Salt and black pepper to taste 2 jars sugar-free marinara sauce 1 cup Italian blend kinds of cheeses 3 tbsp fresh basil, chopped Preheat oven to 400°F.

Directions

Combine the coconut milk and pork rinds in a bowl. Mix in the ground pork, garlic, asiago cheese, Parmesan cheese, eggs, salt, and pepper and stir. Form balls of the mixture and place them in a greased baking pan. Bake in the oven for 20 minutes. Transfer the meatballs to a plate. Pour half of the marinara sauce into the baking pan. Place the meatballs back in the pan and pour in the remaining marinara sauce. Sprinkle with the Italian blend cheeses and drizzle with the olive oil. Cover the pan with foil and put it back in the oven. Bake for 10 minutes. After, remove the foil, and cook for 5 minutes. Once ready, take out the pan and garnish with basil. Serve on a bed of squash spaghetti.

12. Charred Tenderloin with Lemon Chimichurri

Ready in about: 64 minutes | Serves: 4 Per serving: Kcal 388, Fat 18g, Net Carbs 2.1g, Protein 28g

Ingredients

13. Lemon Chimichurri

1 lemon, juiced ¼ cup mint leaves, chopped ¼ cup fresh oregano, chopped 2 cloves garlic, minced ¼ cup olive oil Salt to taste

Pork

1 (4 lb) pork tenderloin Salt and black pepper to taste 1 tbsp olive oil Make the lemon chimichurri to have the flavors incorporate while the pork cooks.

Directions

In a bowl, mix the mint, oregano, and garlic. Then, add the lemon juice, olive oil, and salt, and combine well. Set aside. Preheat the charcoal grill to 450°F, creating a direct heat area and indirect heat area. Rub the pork with olive oil and season with salt and pepper. Place the meat over direct heat and sear for 3 minutes on each side, moving to the indirect heat area. Close the lid and cook for 25 minutes on one side Next, open, turn the meat, and grill for 20 minutes on the other side. Remove the pork from the grill and let it sit for 5 minutes before slicing. Spoon lemon chimichurri over the pork and serve with fresh salad.

14. Pork Goulash with Cauliflower

Ready in about: 15 minutes | Serves: 4 Per serving: Kcal 475, Fat 37g, Net Carbs 4.5g, Protein 44g

Ingredients

1 red bell pepper, chopped 2 tbsp olive oil 1 ½ lb ground pork Salt and black pepper to taste 2 cups cauliflower florets 1 onion, chopped 14 oz canned diced tomatoes ¼ tsp garlic powder 1 tbsp tomato puree

Directions

Heat olive oil in a pan over medium heat. Add in the pork and brown for 5 minutes. Mix in the bell pepper and onion and cook for 4 minutes. Stir in 1 cup water, tomatoes, and cauliflower. Bring to a simmer and cook for 5 minutes. Pour in tomato paste, salt, pepper, and garlic powder and stir for 5 minutes. Serve.

15. Pork Wraps

Ready in about: 40 minutes | Serves: 6 Per serving: Kcal 435, Fat 37g, Net Carbs 2g, Protein 34g

Ingredients 6 bacon slices 2 tbsp fresh parsley, chopped 1 lb pork tenderloin, sliced ⅓ cup ricotta cheese 3 tbsp coconut oil ¼ cup onions, chopped 3 garlic cloves, minced 2 tbsp Parmesan cheese, grated 15 oz canned diced tomatoes ⅓ cup vegetable stock Salt and black pepper to taste ½ tsp Italian seasoning

Directions

Use a meat pounder to flatten the pork pieces. Set the bacon slices on top of each piece and divide the parsley, ricotta cheese, and Parmesan cheese between them. Roll each pork piece and secure it with a toothpick. Set a pan over medium heat and warm oil. Cook the pork rolls until browned. Remove. Add onions and garlic in the pan and cook for 5 minutes. Place in the stock and cook for 3 minutes. Get rid of the toothpicks from the rolls and return to the pan. Stir in pepper, salt, tomatoes, and Italian seasoning. Bring to a boil, reduce the heat, and cook for 20 minutes covered. Split among bowls to serve.

16. Pulled Pork with Avocado

Ready in about: 2 hours 55 minutes | Serves: 6 Per serving: Kcal 567, Fat 42.6g, Net Carbs 4.1g, Protein 42g

Ingredients 2 lb pork shoulder 1 tbsp avocado oil ½ cup vegetable stock 1 tsp taco seasoning 1 avocado, sliced Preheat oven to 350°F.

DirectionsRub the pork with taco seasoning and set in a greased baking dish. Pour in the vegetable stock. Place in the oven, cover with aluminium foil, and cook for 1 hour 45 minutes. Discard the foil and cook for another 10-15 minutes until brown on top. Leave to rest for 15-20 minutes. Shred it with 2 forks. Serve topped with avocado slices.

17. BBQ Pork Pizza with Goat Cheese

Ready in about: 30 minutes | Serves: 4 Per serving: Kcal 344, Fat 24g, Net Carbs 6,5g, Protein 18g

Ingredients 1 low carb pizza bread 1 tbsp olive oil 1 cup Manchego cheese, grated 2 cups leftover pulled pork ½ cup sugar-free BBQ sauce 1 cup goat cheese, crumbled Preheat oven to 400°F.

Directions

Put the pizza bread on a pizza pan. Brush with olive oil and sprinkle the Manchego cheese all over. Mix the pork with BBQ sauce and spread over the cheese. Drop goat cheese on top and bake for 25 minutes until the cheese has melted. Slice the pizza with a cutter and serve.

18. Easy Pork Bistek

(Ready in about 30 minutes | Servings 4) Per serving: 305 Calories; 20.6g Fat; 3.7g Carbs; 22.5g Protein; 0.6g

Ingredients 1 red onion, peeled and chopped 1 garlic clove, minced 2 tablespoons olive oil 1 ½ pounds pork blade steak 1/4 cup dry red wine 1/2 teaspoon salt 1/2 teaspoon freshly ground black pepper 1/2 teaspoon cayenne pepper 1 teaspoon mustard seeds

Directions

In a frying pan, heat 1 tablespoon of the olive oil over a moderate heat. Now, sear the pork steaks for 8 to 9 minutes per side. Pour in a splash of wine to deglaze the pot. Sprinkle with spices and continue to cook for 10 minutes more, adding additional water if necessary; reserve. In the same frying pan, heat the remaining tablespoon of olive oil and cook the onions and garlic until they have softened. Bon appétit!

19. Italian-Style Pork Casserole

(Ready in about 50 minutes | Servings 6) Per serving: 478 Calories; 36g Fat; 4.9g Carbs; 33.5g Protein; 0.3g

Ingredients 1 ¼ pounds ground pork 6 eggs, lightly beaten 2 tablespoons fresh Italian parsley 2 ½ cups almond meal 1 Italian peppers, thinly sliced 1 cup double cream 1/2 teaspoon celery seeds 1 stick butter, melted Salt and pepper, to the taste

Directions Start by preheating your oven to 350 degrees F Thoroughly combine the eggs, almond meal, and melted until well combined. Press the mixture into a lightly oiled baking dish. In a nonstick skillet, cook the ground pork for about 4 minutes, breaking apart with a wide spatula; season with salt and pepper to taste. Add in the remaining ingredients and stir to combine well. Spread this mixture over the crust, using a wide spatula. Bake in the preheated oven at 350 degrees F for about 40 minutes. Let it stand for 10 minutes before slicing. Bon appétit!

20. Roasted Pork Rib Chops

(Ready in about 30 minutes + marinating time | Servings 4) Per serving: 452 Calories; 34.8g Fat; 4.7g Carbs; 26.3g

Ingredients

4 (2-1 1/2"-thick) pork bone-in pork rib chops 1 teaspoon mustard seeds 2 tablespoons fresh lime juice 1/2 teaspoon celery salt 1/2 teaspoon freshly ground black pepper 1 garlic clove 2 tablespoons butter, room temperature 1 cup leeks, sliced 2 carrots, sliced 1 celery stalk, diced

Directions

Place the pork, mustard seeds, fresh lime juice, celery salt, salt, pepper, and garlic in a ceramic dish. Cover and let them marinate in your refrigerator for about 3 hours. In an oven-safe skillet, melt the butter over medium-high heat. Sear the pork cutlets until bottom side is golden brown, about 2 minutes. Flip them over and cook on other side about 2 minutes. Repeat the process, turning about every 1 to 2 minutes, until an instant-read thermometer inserted into the thickest part registers 150 degrees F. Add in the leeks, carrots, and celery and continue to cook, partially covered, for 5 minutes more. Transfer the skillet to the oven and roast the pork with the vegetables for about 10 minutes. Bon appétit!

21. Mom's Signature Pork Meatloaf

(Ready in about 45 minutes | Servings 6) Per serving: 251 Calories; 7.9g Fat; 4.5g Carbs; 34.6g Protein; 1.4g

Ingredients

1 cup tomato puree, no sugar added 1 ½ tablespoons Swerve 1 tablespoon champagne vinegar 1/2 teaspoon dried rosemary 1 teaspoon fresh coriander 1/3 cup almond meal 1 large egg Sea salt and ground black pepper 1 teaspoon celery seeds 1 ½ pounds ground pork 1/4 cup pork rinds, crushed 1 large onion, chopped 2 cloves garlic, finely minced

Directions

In a mixing dish, thoroughly combine the almond meal, egg, salt, black pepper, celery seeds, ground pork, pork rinds, onion, and garlic. Press the meatloaf mixture into a lightly greased loaf pan. In a saucepan, cook the remaining ingredients until the sauce has thickened and reduced slightly. Spread the sauce evenly over the top of your meatloaf. Roast in the preheated oven at 365 degrees F for 35 minutes. Place under the preheated broiler for 5 to 6 minutes. Bon appétit!

22. Pork Rib Soup with Avocado

(Ready in about 20 minutes | Servings 6) Per serving: 423 Calories; 31.8g Fat; 6g Carbs; 25.9g Protein; 3.2g

Ingredients

1 ¼ pounds pork spare ribs, boneless and cut into chunks 2 tablespoons butter, room temperature Sea salt and ground black pepper, to taste A pinch of dried Mexican oregano 2 vine-ripened tomatoes, undrained 1 celery, chopped 1 onion, peeled and chopped 1 teaspoon garlic, crushed 1 teaspoon habanero pepper, seeded and minced 3 cups beef broth, less-sodium 1/4 cup fresh coriander, roughly chopped 1 medium-sized avocado, pitted and sliced

Directions

Melt the butter in a heavy-bottomed pot over a moderate heat. Sauté the onion, garlic, pepper and celery approximately 3 minutes. Then, sear the pork for 4 to 5 minutes, stirring continuously to ensure even cooking. Add in the broth, salt, black pepper, oregano, tomatoes, and coriander. Continue to simmer, partially covered, for about 12 minutes. Bon appétit!

23. Creamed Pork Soup

(Ready in about 25 minutes | Servings 4) Per serving: 490 Calories; 44g Fat; 6.1g Carbs; 24.3g Protein; 2.2g Fiber

Ingredients

3/4 pound pork chops, cubed 2 tomatoes, pureed 1 cup double cream 1/2 teaspoon Tabasco sauce 1 tablespoon chicken bouillon granules 4 cups water 2 tablespoons butter, melted 1 white onion, chopped 1 celery stalk, chopped 1 carrot, chopped Seasoned salt and freshly cracked black pepper, to taste 1/2 teaspoon red pepper flakes 1/2 cup avocado, pitted, peeled and diced

Directions

In a soup pot, melt the butter over medium-high heat. Cook the onion, celery, and carrot until tender and fragrant or about 6 minutes. Heat the remaining tablespoon of butter and sear the pork for 4 to 5 minutes, stirring periodically to ensure even cooking. Add in the water, pureed tomatoes, chicken bouillon granules, salt, black pepper, and red paper flakes, salt, and pepper. Partially cover and continue to simmer for 10 to 12 minutes. Fold in the double cream and Tabasco sauce. Let it simmer for 5 minutes until cooked through .Bon appétit!

24. Saucy Boston Butt

(Ready in about 1 hour 20 minutes | Servings 8) Per serving: 369 Calories; 20.2g Fat; 2.9g Carbs; 41.3g Protein; 0.7g Fiber

Ingredients

1 tablespoon lard, room temperature 2 pounds Boston butt, cubed Salt and freshly ground pepper 1/2 teaspoon mustard powder A bunch of spring onions, chopped 2 garlic cloves, minced 1/2 tablespoon ground cardamom 2 tomatoes, pureed 1 bell pepper, deveined and chopped 1 jalapeno pepper, deveined and finely chopped 1/2 cup unsweetened coconut milk 2 cups chicken bone broth

Directions

In a wok, melt the lard over moderate heat. Season the pork belly with salt, pepper and mustard powder. Sear the pork for 8 to 10 minutes, stirring periodically to ensure even cooking; set aside, keeping it warm. In the same wok, sauté the spring onions, garlic, and cardamom. Spoon the sautéed vegetables along with the reserved pork into the slow cooker. Add in the remaining ingredients, cover with the lid and cook for 1 hour 10 minutes over low heat. Bon appétit!

25. Pork in Blue Cheese Sauce

(Ready in about 30 minutes | Servings 6) Per serving: 348 Calories; 18.9g Fat; 1.9g Carbs; 40.3g Protein; 0.3g Fiber

Ingredients

2 pounds pork center cut loin roast, boneless and cut into 6 pieces 1 tablespoon coconut aminos 6 ounces blue cheese 1/3 cup heavy cream 1/3 cup port wine 1/3 cup roasted vegetable broth, preferably homemade 1 teaspoon dried hot chile flakes 1 teaspoon dried rosemary 1 tablespoon lard 1 shallot, chopped 2 garlic cloves, chopped Salt and freshly cracked black peppercorns, to taste

Directions

Rub each piece of the pork with salt, black peppercorns, and rosemary. Melt the lard in a saucepan over a moderately high flame. Sear the pork on all sides about 15 minutes; set aside. Cook the shallot and garlic until they've softened. Add in port wine to scrape up any brown bits from the bottom. Reduce the heat to medium-low and add in the remaining ingredients; continue to simmer until the sauce has thickened and reduced. Bon appétit!

26. Mediterranean-Style Cheesy Pork Loin

(Ready in about 25 minutes | Servings 4) Per serving: 476 Calories; 35.3g Fat; 6.2g Carbs; 31.1g Protein; 1.4g Fiber

Ingredients 1 pound pork loin, cut into 1-inch-thick pieces 1 teaspoon Mediterranean seasoning mix Salt and pepper, to taste 1 onion, sliced 1 teaspoon fresh garlic, smashed 2 tablespoons black olives, pitted and sliced 2 tablespoons balsamic vinegar 1/2 cup Romano cheese, grated 2 tablespoons butter, room temperature 1 tablespoon curry paste 1 cup roasted vegetable broth 1 tablespoon oyster sauce

Directions

In a frying pan, melt the butter over a moderately high heat. Once hot, cook the pork until browned on all sides; season with salt and black pepper and set aside. In the pan drippings, cook the onion and garlic for 4 to 5 minutes or until they've softened. Add in the Mediterranean seasoning mix, curry paste, and vegetable broth. Continue to cook until the sauce has thickened and reduced slightly or about 10 minutes. Add in the remaining ingredients along with the reserved pork. Top with cheese and cook for 10 minutes longer or until cooked through.Enjoy!

27. Oven-Roasted Spare Ribs

(Ready in about 3 hour 40 minutes + marinating time | Servings 6) Per serving: 385 Calories; 29g Fat; 1.8g Carbs; 28.3g Protein; 0.1g Fiber

Ingredients 2 pounds spare ribs 1 garlic clove, minced 1 teaspoon dried marjoram 1 lime, halved Salt and ground black pepper, to taste

Directions

Toss all ingredients in a ceramic dish. Cover and let it refrigerate for 5 to 6 hours. Roast the foil-wrapped ribs in the preheated oven at 275 degrees F degrees for about 3 hours 30 minutes. Bon appétit!

28. Peanut Butter Pork Stir-Fry

Ready in about: 23 minutes | Serves: 4 Per serving: Kcal 571, Fat 49g, Net Carbs 1g, Protein 22.5g

Ingredients

2 tbsp ghee 2 lb pork loin, cut into strips Pink salt to taste 2 tsp ginger-garlic paste ¼ cup chicken broth 5 tbsp peanut butter, softened 2 cups mixed stir-fry vegetables ½ tsp chili pepper

Directions Melt the ghee in a wok over high heat. Rub the pork with salt, chili pepper, and ginger-garlic paste. Place it into the wok and cook for 6 minutes until no longer pink. Mix peanut butter and broth until smooth. Pour in the wok and stir for 6 minutes. Add in the mixed veggies and simmer for 5 minutes. Adjust the taste with salt and black pepper and spoon the stir-fry to a side of cilantro cauli rice.

29. Pork Lettuce Cups

Ready in about: 20 minutes | Serves: 6 Per serving: Kcal 311, Fat 24.3g, Net Carbs 1g, Protein 19g

Ingredients

2 lb ground pork 1 tbsp ginger-garlic paste Pink salt and black pepper to taste 3 tbsp butter Leaves from 1 head Iceberg lettuce 2 green onions, chopped 1 red bell pepper, chopped ½ cucumber, finely chopped ½ tsp cayenne pepper

Directions

Melt the butter in a pan over medium heat. Rub the pork with ginger-garlic paste, salt, pepper, and cayenne pepper and add it to the pan. Cook for 10 minutes until the pork is no longer pink. Remove and let it cool. Pat the lettuce leaves dry with paper towels. Spoon two to three tablespoons of the pork mixture in each leaf. Top with green onions, bell pepper, and cucumber. Serve with soy drizzling sauce.

30. Pork & Mushroom Bake

Ready in about: 1 hour 15 minutes | Serves: 6 Per serving: Kcal 403, Fat: 32.6g, Net Carbs: 8g, Protein: 19.4g

Ingredients

1 onion, chopped 2 (10.5-oz) cans mushroom soup 6 pork chops ½ cup sliced mushrooms Salt and black pepper to taste Preheat oven to 370°F.

Directions

Season the pork with salt and pepper. Place on a baking dish. Combine the mushroom soup, mushrooms, and onion in a bowl and stir. Pour it over the pork. Bake for 45 minutes.

31. Pork Chops with Mint & Parsley Pesto

Ready in about: 3 hours 10 minutes | Serves: 4 Per serving: Kcal 567, Fat 40g, Net Carbs 5.5g, Protein 37g

Ingredients

1 cup parsley 1 cup mint 1 ½ onions, chopped ⅓ cup pistachios, chopped 3 tbsp avocado oil Salt to taste 4 pork chops 2 garlic cloves, minced 1 lemon, juiced and zested

DirectionsIn a food processor, combine the parsley with avocado oil, mint, pistachios, salt, lemon zest, and half of the onions. Rub the pork with this mixture, place In a bowl, and refrigerate for 1 hour while covered. Remove the chops and set them to a baking dish. Top with the remaining onions and garlic. Sprinkle with lemon juice. Pour in 1 cup of water. Bake for 2 hours in the oven at 250°F. Serve warm.

32. Bacon Smothered Pork Chops

Ready in about: 25 minutes | Serves: 6 Per serving: Kcal 435, Fat 37g, Net Carbs 3g, Protein 22g

Ingredients

6 strips bacon, chopped 6 pork chops Pink salt and black pepper to taste 2 sprigs fresh thyme ¼ cup chicken broth ½ cup heavy cream

Directions

Cook bacon in a large skillet on medium heat for 5 minutes. Remove with a slotted spoon onto a paper towel-lined plate to soak up excess fat. Season the pork chops with salt and black pepper and brown in the bacon fat for 4 minutes on each side. Remove to the bacon plate. Stir the thyme, chicken broth, and heavy cream in the skillet and simmer for 5 minutes. Return the chops and bacon and cook further for another 2 minutes. Serve chops with a generous ladle of sauce.

33. Pancetta & Kale Pork Sausages

Ready in about: 30 minutes | Serves: 4 Per serving: Kcal 386, Fat 29g, Net Carbs 5.4g, Protein2 1g

Ingredients

2 cups kale 4 cups chicken broth 2 tbsp olive oil 1 cup heavy cream 3 pancetta slices, chopped ½ lb radishes, chopped 2 garlic cloves, minced Salt and black pepper to taste ½ tsp red pepper flakes 1 onion, chopped 1 ½ lb hot pork sausage, chopped

Directions

Warm the olive oil in a pot over medium heat. Stir in garlic, onion, pancetta, and sausage and cook for 5 minutes. Pour in the broth, radishes, and kale and simmer for 10 minutes. Sprinkle with salt, red pepper flakes, and black pepper. Add in the heavy cream, stir, and cook for about 5 minutes. Serve.

34. Juicy Pork Medallions

Ready in about: 30 minutes | Serves: 4 Per serving: Kcal 325, Fat 18g, Net Carbs 6g, Protein 36g

Ingredients

1 lb pork tenderloin, cut into medallions 2 onions, chopped 6 bacon slices, chopped ½ cup vegetable stock

DirectionsSet a pan over medium heat. Add in the bacon and cook until crispy, about 5 minutes; remove to a plate. Add onions to the pan and cook for 3 minutes; set aside. Add the pork medallions to the pan Brown for 3 minutes on each side, turn, and reduce the heat. Add in the vegetable stock and cook for 10 minutes. Return the bacon and onions to the pan and cook for 1 minute. Serve warm.

35. Lemon Pork Chops with Buttered Brussels Sprouts

Ready in about: 35 minutes | Serves: 6 Per serving: Kcal 549, Fat 48g, Net Carbs 2g, Protein 26g

Ingredients

3 tbsp lemon juice 3 cloves garlic, pureed 2 tbsp olive oil 6 pork loin chops 1 tbsp butter 1 lb Brussels sprouts, trimmed, halved 2 tbsp white wine Salt and black pepper to taste Preheat oven to 400°F.

Directions

Mix the lemon juice, garlic, salt, black pepper, and oil in a bowl. Brush the pork with the mixture. Place in a baking sheet and brown in the oven for 15 minutes, turning once. Remove. Melt butter in a small wok and cook the Brussels sprouts for 5 minutes until tender. Drizzle with white wine, sprinkle with salt and black pepper, and cook for another 5 minutes. Serve them with the chops.

36. Greek Pork with Olives

Ready in about: 35 minutes | Serves: 4 Per serving: Kcal 415, Fat 25.2g, Net Carbs 2.2g, Protein 36g

Ingredients

4 pork chops, bone-in Salt and black pepper to taste 2 garlic cloves, minced ½ cup Kalamata olives, pitted, sliced 2 tbsp olive oil 1 cup vegetable broth Season pork chops with black pepper and salt.

Directions

Add them to a roasting pan. Add in garlic, olives, olive oil, and vegetable broth. Roast in the oven for 10 minutes at 425°F. Serve warm.

37. Pork Nachos

Ready in about: 15 minutes | Serves: 4 Per serving: Kcal 452, Fat 25g, Net Carbs 9.3g, Protein 22g

Ingredients

1 bag low carb tortilla chips 2 cups leftover pulled pork 1 red bell pepper, chopped 1 red onion, diced 2 cups Monterey Jack cheese, grated Preheat oven to 350°F.

Directions

Arrange the chips on a baking pan, scatter pork over, followed by red bell pepper and onion, and sprinkle with the cheese. Place the pan in the oven and cook for 10 minutes until the cheese has melted. Allow cooling for 3 minutes and serve.

38. Balsamic Grilled Pork Chops

Ready in about: 20 minutes + marinating time | Serves: 6 Per serving: Kcal 418, Fat 26.8g, Net Carbs 1.5g, Protein 38g

Ingredients

6 pork loin chops, boneless 1 tbsp erythritol ¼ cup balsamic vinegar 3 cloves garlic, minced ¼ cup olive oil Salt and black pepper to taste Put the pork in a plastic bag.

Directions

In a bowl, mix the erythritol, balsamic vinegar, garlic, olive oil, salt, pepper, and pour the mixture over the pork. Seal the bag, shake it, and place it in the refrigerator for 2 hours. Preheat the grill to medium heat, remove the pork when ready, and grill covered for 10 minutes on each side. Remove and let sit for 4 minutes. Serve with sautéed parsnips.

39. Pork Stew with Bacon & Cauliflower

Ready in about: 40 minutes | Serves: 6 Per serving: Kcal 331, Fat 14.2g, Net Carbs 2.9g, Protein 43.8g

Ingredients

2 lb pork tenderloin, cubed 2 cups chicken broth 3 tbsp olive oil 1 onion, chopped Salt and black pepper to taste 2 garlic cloves, minced 1 cup canned diced tomatoes 1 cup bacon, chopped 1 head cauliflower, cut into florets

Directions

Warm the olive oil in a saucepan over medium heat. Add in the bacon, pork, onion, and garlic and sauté for 3-4 minutes until the onion is tender. Pour in the chicken stock and tomatoes and simmer for 20-25 minutes. Add in the cauliflower and cook for 10 more minutes. Season with salt and pepper. Serve warm.

40. Beef Mushroom Meatloaf

Ready in about: 1 hour and 15 minutes | Serves: 12 Per serving: Kcal 294, Fat: 19g, Net Carbs: 6g, Protein: 23g

Ingredients 3 pounds ground beef ½ cup chopped onions ½ cup almond flour 2 garlic cloves, minced 1 cup sliced mushrooms 3 eggs ¼ tsp pepper 2 tbsp chopped parsley ¼ cup chopped bell peppers ⅓ cup grated Parmesan cheese 1 tsp balsamic vinegar 1 tsp salt Glaze 2 cups balsamic vinegar 1 tbsp sweetener 2 tbsp sugar-free ketchup

DirectionsCombine all meatloaf ingredients in a large bowl. Press this mixture into a greased loaf pans. Bake in the oven for 30 minutes at 370°F. Combine all the glaze ingredients in a saucepan over medium heat. Simmer for 20 minutes until the glaze is thickened. Pour ¼ cup of the glaze over the meatloaf. Save the extra for future use. Put the meatloaf back in the oven and cook for 20 more minutes.

41. Beef & Cheddar Stuffed Eggplants

Ready in about: 30 minutes | Serves: 4 Per serving: Kcal 574, Fat 27.5g, Net Carbs 9.8g, Protein 61,8g

Ingredients

2 eggplants 2 tbsp olive oil 1 ½ lb ground beef 1 medium red onion, chopped 1 roasted red pepper, chopped Pink salt and black pepper to taste 1 cup yellow cheddar cheese, grated 2 tbsp dill, chopped Preheat oven to 350°F.

DirectionsLay the eggplants on a flat surface, trim off the ends, and cut in half lengthwise. Scoop out the pulp from each half to make shells. Chop the pulp. Heat oil in a skillet over medium heat. Add the ground beef, red onion, pimiento, and eggplant pulp and season with salt and pepper. Cook for 6 minutes while stirring to break up lumps until beef is no longer pink. Spoon the beef into the eggplant shells and sprinkle with cheddar cheese. Place on a greased baking sheet and cook to Melt the cheese for 15 minutes until eggplant is tender. Serve warm topped with dill.

42. Melt-in-Your-Mouth Ribs

(Ready in about 4 hours 30 minutes | Servings 4) Per serving: 412 Calories; 14g Fat; 4.3g Carbs; 43.3g Protein; 0.7g

Ingredients 1 ½ pounds spare ribs 1 tablespoon olive oil, at room temperature 2 cloves garlic, chopped 1 Italian pepper, chopped Salt and black peppercorns, to taste 1/2 teaspoon ground cumin 2 bay leaves A bunch of green onions, chopped 3/4 cup beef bone broth, preferably homemade 2 teaspoons erythritol

Directions Heat the olive oil in a saucepan over medium-high heat. Sear the ribs for 6 to 7 minutes on each side. Whisk the broth, erythritol, garlic, Italian pepper, green onions, salt, pepper, and cumin until well combined. Place the spare ribs in your crock pot; pour in the pepper/broth mixture. Add in the bay leaves. Cook for about 4 hours on Low setting.

43. Old-Fashioned Stew with Pork Butt

Butt (Ready in about 25 minutes | Servings 4) Per serving: 295 Calories; 15.6g Fat; 6.3g Carbs; 17.3g Protein; 1.1g

Ingredients

3/4 pound boneless pork butt, cubed 1 ½ cups vegetable stock 1 tablespoon lard, room temperature 1 teaspoon Serrano pepper, deveined and minced 2 garlic cloves, minced 1/2 teaspoon ground cloves 1 yellow onion, chopped 1 carrot, chopped 1 tablespoon fresh coriander, chopped 2 ounces cream cheese, full-fat Himalayan salt and ground black pepper, to taste

Directions

Melt the lard in a soup pot over medium-high heat. Now, sauté the onion, carrot, and Serrano pepper for about 4 minutes or until tender and fragrant. Add in the boneless pork butt and cook for a father 5 to 6 minutes, stirring continuously to ensure even cooking. Add in the garlic, vegetable stock, ground cloves, salt, black pepper, and coriander; bring to a rapid boil. Now, reduce the temperature to medium-low. Cook for 15 to 20 minutes or until everything is thoroughly cooked. Bon appétit!

44. Pork and Carrot Mini Muffins

(Ready in about 35 minutes | Servings 6) Per serving: 303 Calories; 17g Fat; 6.2g Carbs; 29.6g Protein; 1.7g

Ingredients 1 egg, whisked 1 ounce envelope onion soup mix Kosher salt and ground black pepper, to taste 2 cloves of garlic, minced 1 cup carrots, shredded 1 cup tomato puree 1 tablespoon coconut aminos 1 tablespoon stone-ground mustard 1 ½ teaspoons dry basil 1 cup Romano cheese, grated 1 pound pork, ground 1/2 pound turkey, ground

Directions In a mixing bowl, combine all ingredients until everything is well incorporated. Press the mixture into a lightly-oiled muffin tin. Bake in the preheated oven at 355 degrees F for 30 to 33 minutes; let it cool slightly before unmolding and serving. Bon appétit!

45. Creole-Style Pork Shank

(Ready in about 30 minutes + marinating time | Servings 6) Per serving: 335 Calories; 24.3g Fat; 0.8g Carbs; 26.4g Protein; 0.4g

Ingredients 1 ½ pounds pork shank, cut into 6 serving portions 1 tablespoon Creole seasoning A few drops of liquid smoke Salt and cayenne pepper, to taste 3 teaspoons vegetable oil 2 clove garlic, minced 1 ½ tablespoons coconut aminos

Directions Blend the salt, cayenne pepper, vegetable oil, garlic, liquid smoke, Creole seasoning, and coconut aminos until you get a uniform and creamy mixture. Massage the pork shanks on all sides with the prepared rub mixture. Let it marinate for about 2 hours in your refrigerator. Grill for about 20 minutes until cooked through. Enjoy!

46. Rich Pork and Bacon Meatloaf

(Ready in about 1 hour 10 minutes | Servings 6) Per serving: 396 Calories; 24.1g Fat; 5.1g Carbs; 38.1g Protein; 0.5g

Ingredients

1 ¼ pounds ground pork 1/2 pound pork sausage, broken up 6 strips bacon 2 garlic cloves, finely minced 1 teaspoon celery seeds Salt and cayenne pepper, to taste 1 bunch coriander, roughly chopped 1 egg, beaten 2 ounces half-and-half 1 teaspoon lard 1 medium-sized leek, chopped

Directions Melt the lard in a frying pan over medium-high heat. Cook the leek and garlic until they have softened or about 3 minutes. Add in the ground pork and sausage; cook until it is no longer pink, about 3 minutes. Add in the half-and-half, celery seeds, salt, cayenne pepper, coriander, and egg. Press the mixture into a loaf pan. Place the bacon strips on top of your meatloaf and bake at 390 degrees F about 55 minutes. Bon appétit!

47. Pork Cutlets with Kale

(Ready in about 25 minutes + marinating time | Servings 6) Per serving: 234 Calories; 11g Fat; 2g Carbs; 29.8g Protein; 0.9g

Ingredients

Sea salt and ground black pepper, to taste 2 teaspoons olive oil 1/4 cup port wine 2 garlic cloves, smashed 2 tablespoons oyster sauce 2 tablespoons fresh lime juice 1 medium leek, sliced 2 bell peppers, chopped 2 cups kale 1 ½ pounds pork cutlets

Directions

Sprinkle the pork with salt and black pepper. Then, make the marinade by whisking 1 teaspoon of olive oil, wine, garlic, oyster sauce, and lime juice. Let the pork marinate for about 2 hours in your refrigerator Heat the remaining teaspoon of olive oil in a frying pan. Fry the leek and bell peppers for 4 to 5 minutes, stirring continuously, until they have softened slightly; set aside. In the same pan, sear the pork along with the marinade until browned on all sides. Stir the reserved vegetables into the frying pan along with the kale. Continue to cook for 5 to 6 minutes more. Bon appétit!

48. Cheesy Chinese-Style Pork

(Ready in about 20 minutes | Servings 6) Per serving: 424 Calories; 29.4g Fat; 3.8g Carbs; 34.2g Protein; 0.6g Fiber

Ingredients

1 tablespoon sesame oil 1 ½ pounds pork shoulder, cut into strips Himalayan salt and freshly ground black pepper, to taste 1/2 teaspoon cayenne pepper 1/2 cup shallots, roughly chopped 2 bell peppers, sliced 1/4 cup cream of onion soup 1/2 teaspoon Sriracha sauce 1 tablespoon tahini (sesame butter) 1 tablespoon soy sauce 4 ounces gouda cheese, cut into small pieces

Directions

Heat he sesame oil in a wok over a moderately high flame. Stir-fry the pork strips for 3 to 4 minutes or until just browned on all sides. Add in the spices, shallots and bell peppers and continue to cook for a further 4 minutes. Stir in the cream of onion soup, Sriracha, sesame butter, and soy sauce; continue to cook for 3 to 4 minutes more. Top with the cheese and continue to cook until the cheese has melted.

49. Breakfast Muffins with Ground Pork

(Ready in about 25 minutes | Servings 6) Per serving: 330 Calories; 30.3g Fat; 2.3g Carbs; 19g Protein; 1.2g Fiber

Ingredients

1 stick butter 3 large eggs, lightly beaten 2 tablespoons full-fat milk 1/2 teaspoon ground cardamom 3 ½ cups almond flour 2 tablespoons flaxseed meal 1 teaspoon baking powder 2 cups ground pork Salt and pepper, to your liking 1/2 teaspoon dried basil

Directions

In the preheated frying pan, cook the ground pork until the juices run clear, approximately 5 minutes. Add in the remaining ingredients and stir until well combined. Spoon the mixture into lightly greased muffin cups. Bake in the preheated oven at 365 degrees F for about 17 minutes. Allow your muffins to cool down before unmolding and storing. Bon appétit!

50. Brie-Stuffed Meatballs

(Ready in about 25 minutes | Servings 5) Per serving: 302 Calories; 17.3g Fat; 1.9g Carbs; 33.4g Protein; 0.3g Fiber

Ingredients

2 eggs, beaten 1 pound ground pork 1/3 cup double cream 1 tablespoon fresh parsley Kosher salt and ground black pepper 1 teaspoon dried rosemary 10 (1-inch) cubes of brie cheese 2 tablespoons scallions, minced 2 cloves garlic, minced

Directions

Mix all ingredients, except for the brie cheese, until everything is well incorporated. Roll the mixture into 10 patties; place a piece of cheese in the center of each patty and roll into a ball. Roast in the preheated oven at 380 degrees F for about 20 minutes. Bon appétit!

POULTRY

51. Autumn Chicken Soup with Root Vegetables

(Ready in about 25 minutes | Servings 4) Per serving: 342 Calories; 22.4g Fat; 6.3g Carbs; 25.2g Protein; 1.3g Fiber

Ingredients

4 cups chicken broth 1 cup full-fat milk 1 cup double cream 1/2 cup turnip, chopped 2 chicken drumsticks, boneless and cut into small pieces Salt and pepper, to taste 1 tablespoon butter 1 teaspoon garlic, finely minced 1 carrot, chopped 1/2 parsnip, chopped 1/2 celery 1 whole egg

Directions Melt the butter in a heavy-bottomed pot over medium-high heat; sauté the garlic until aromatic or about 1 minute. Add in the vegetables and continue to cook until they've softened. Add in the chicken and cook until it is no longer pink for about 4 minutes. Season with salt and pepper. Pour in the chicken broth, milk, and heavy cream and bring it to a boil. Reduce the heat to. Partially cover and continue to simmer for 20 to 25 minutes longer. Afterwards, fold the beaten egg and stir until it is well incorporated.Bon appétit!

52. Breaded Chicken Fillets

(Ready in about 30 minutes | Servings 4) Per serving: 367 Calories; 16.9g Fat; 6g Carbs; 43g Protein; 0.7g Fiber

Ingredients

1 pound chicken fillets 3 bell peppers, quartered lengthwise 1/3 cup Romano cheese 2 teaspoons olive oil 1 garlic clove, minced Kosher salt and ground black pepper, to taste 1/3 cup crushed pork rinds

Directions Start by preheating your oven to 410 degrees F. Mix the crushed pork rinds, Romano cheese, olive oil and minced garlic. Dredge the chicken into this mixture. Place the chicken in a lightly greased baking dish. Season with salt and black pepper to taste. Scatter the peppers around the chicken and bake in the preheated oven for 20 to 25 minutes or until thoroughly cooked. Enjoy!

53. Greek-Style Saucy Chicken Drumettes

(Ready in about 50 minutes | Servings 6) Per serving: 333 Calories; 20.2g Fat; 2g Carbs; 33.5g Protein; 0.2g Fiber

Ingredients

1 ½ pounds chicken drumettes 1/2 cup port wine 1/2 cup onions, chopped 2 garlic cloves, minced 1 teaspoon tzatziki spice mix 1 cup double cream 2 tablespoons butter Sea salt and crushed mixed peppercorns, to season

Directions

Melt the butter in an oven-proof skillet over a moderate heat; then, cook the chicken for about 8 minutes. Add in the onions, garlic, wine, tzatziki spice mix, double cream, salt, and pepper. Bake in the preheated oven at 390 degrees F for 35 to 40 minutes (a meat thermometer should register 165 degrees F).Enjoy!

54. Herbed Chicken Breasts

(Ready in about 40 minutes | Servings 8) Per serving: 306 Calories; 17.8g Fat; 3.1g Carbs; 31.7g Protein; 0.2g Fiber

Ingredients

4 chicken breasts, skinless and boneless 1 Italian pepper, deveined and thinly sliced 10 black olives, pitted 1 ½ cups vegetable broth 2 garlic cloves, pressed 2 tablespoons olive oil 1 tablespoon Old Sub Sailor Salt, to taste

Directions Rub the chicken with the garlic and Old Sub Sailor; salt to taste. Heat the oil in a frying pan over a moderately high heat. Sear the chicken until it is browned on all sides, about 5 minutes. Add in the pepper, olives, and vegetable broth and bring it to boil. Reduce the heat simmer and continue to cook, partially covered, for 30 to 35 minutes. Bon appétit!

55. Festive Turkey Rouladen

(Ready in about 30 minutes | Servings 5) Per serving: 286 Calories; 9.7g Fat; 6.9g Carbs; 39.9g Protein; 0.3g Fiber

Ingredients 2 pounds turkey fillet, marinated and cut into 10 pieces 10 strips prosciutto 1/2 teaspoon chili powder 1 teaspoon marjoram 1 sprig rosemary, finely chopped 2 tablespoons dry white wine 1 teaspoon garlic, finely minced 1 ½ tablespoons butter, room temperature 1 tablespoon Dijon mustard Sea salt and freshly ground black pepper, to your liking

Directions Start by preheating your oven to 430 degrees F. Pat the turkey dry and cook in hot butter for about 3 minutes per side. Add in the mustard, chili powder, marjoram, rosemary, wine, and garlic. Continue to cook for 2 minutes more. Wrap each turkey piece into one prosciutto strip and secure with toothpicks. Roast in the preheated oven for about 30 minutes.Bon appétit!

56. Chinese Bok Choy and Turkey Soup

(Ready in about 40 minutes | Servings 8) Per serving: 211 Calories; 11.8g Fat; 3.1g Carbs; 23.7g Protein; 0.9g Fiber

Ingredients

1/2 pound baby Bok choy, sliced into quarters lengthwise 2 pounds turkey carcass 1 tablespoon olive oil 1/2 cup leeks, chopped 1 celery rib, chopped 2 carrots, sliced 6 cups turkey stock Himalayan salt and black pepper, to taste

Directions

In a heavy-bottomed pot, heat the olive oil until sizzling. Once hot, sauté the celery, carrots, leek and Bok choy for about 6 minutes. Add the salt, pepper, turkey, and stock; bring to a boil. Turn the heat to simmer. Continue to cook, partially covered, for about 35 minutes.Bon appétit!

57. Spicy Breakfast Sausage

(Ready in about 15 minutes | Servings 4) Per serving: 156 Calories; 4.2g Fat; 4.1g Carbs; 16.2g Protein; 2.1g Fiber

Ingredients

4 chicken sausages, sliced 1 chili pepper, minced 1 cup shallots, diced 1/4 cup dry white wine 2 teaspoons lard, room temperature 1 teaspoon garlic, minced 2 Spanish peppers, deveined and chopped 2 tablespoons fresh coriander, minced 2 teaspoons balsamic vinegar 1 cup pureed tomatoes

Directions

In a frying pan, warm the lard over moderately high flame. Then, sear the sausage until well browned on all sides; add in the remaining ingredients and stir to combine. Allow it to simmer over low heat for 10 minutes or until thickened slightly.Enjoy!

58. Chicken Fajitas with Peppers and Cheese

(Ready in about 15 minutes | Servings 4) Per serving: 301 Calories; 11.4g Fat; 5.2g Carbs; 37.9g Protein; 2.2g Fiber

Ingredients1 Habanero pepper, deveined and chopped 4 banana peppers, deveined and chopped 1 teaspoon Mexican seasoning blend 1 tablespoon avocado oil 2 garlic cloves, minced 1 cup onions, chopped 1 pound chicken, ground 1/3 cup dry sherry Salt and black pepper, to taste 1/2 cup Cotija cheese, shredded

Directions In a skillet, heat the avocado oil over a moderate flame. Sauté the garlic, onions, and peppers until they are tender and aromatic or about 5 minutes. Fold in the ground chicken and continue to cook until the juices run clear. Add in the dry sherry, Mexican seasonings, salt and pepper. Continue to cook for 5 to 6 minutes more or until cooked through.Enjoy!

59. Chicken Breasts with Mustard Sauce

(Ready in about 25 minutes | Servings 4) Per serving: 415 Calories; 33.2g Fat; 4.5g Carbs; 24.6g Protein; 1.1g Fiber

Ingredients 1/4 cup vegetable broth 1/2 cup heavy whipped cream 1/2 cup onions, chopped 2 garlic cloves, minced 1/4 cup Marsala wine 2 tablespoons brown mustard 1/2 cup fresh parsley, roughly chopped 1 tablespoon olive oil 1 pound chicken breasts, butterflied Salt and pepper, to taste

Directions

Heat the oil in a frying pan over a moderate flame. Cook the chicken breasts until no longer pink or about 6 minutes; season with salt and pepper to taste and reserve. Cook the onion and garlic until it is fragrant or about 5 minutes. Add in the wine to scrape the bits that may be stuck to the bottom of your frying pan. Pour in the broth and bring to boil. Fold in the double cream, mustard, and parsley.Bon appétit!

60. Easy Turkey Meatballs

(Ready in about 20 minutes | Servings 4) Per serving: 244 Calories; 13.7g Fat; 5g Carbs; 27.6g Protein; 2.2g Fiber

Ingredients For the Meatballs: 1/3 cup Colby cheese, freshly grated 3/4 pound ground turkey 1/3 teaspoon Five-spice powder 1 egg For the Sauce: 1 1/3 cups water 1/3 cup champagne vinegar 2 tablespoons soy sauce 1/2 cup Swerve 1/2 cup tomato sauce, no sugar added 1/2 teaspoon paprika 1/3 teaspoon guar gum

Directions Thoroughly combine all ingredients for the meatballs. Roll the mixture into balls and sear them until browned on all sides. In a saucepan, mix all of the sauce ingredients and cook until the sauce has thickened, whisking continuously. Fold the meatballs into the sauce and continue to cook, partially covered, for about 10 minutes.Bon appétit!

61. Chicken Drumettes with Leeks and Herbs

(Ready in about 30 minutes | Servings 4) Per serving: 165 Calories; 9.8g Fat; 4.7g Carbs; 12.4g Protein; 1.3g Fiber

Ingredients 4 chicken drumettes 2 tomatoes, crushed 2 tablespoons lard, room temperature 1 tablespoon coconut aminos 1 teaspoon dried marjoram 2 thyme sprigs Salt and pepper, to taste 2 cloves garlic, minced 1/2 teaspoon fennel seeds 1 cup chicken bone broth 1/2 cup leeks, chopped 1 celery rib, sliced

Directions Melt the lard in a frying pan over a moderate heat. Sprinkle the chicken with salt and pepper to taste. Then, fry the chicken until no longer pink or about 8 minutes; set aside. In the same frying pan, cook the leeks, celery rib, and garlic for about 5 minutes, stirring continuously. Reduce the heat to medium-low; add the remaining ingredients along with the reserved chicken drumettes. Let it simmer for about 20 minutes.Enjoy!

62. Roasted Chicken with Cashew Pesto

(Ready in about 35 minutes | Servings 4) Per serving: 580 Calories; 44.8g Fat; 5g Carbs; 38.7g Protein; 1g Fiber

Ingredients

1 cup leeks, chopped 1 pound chicken legs, skinless Salt and ground black pepper, to taste 1/2 teaspoon red pepper flakes For the Cashew-Basil Pesto: 1/2 cup cashews 2 garlic cloves, minced 1/2 cup fresh basil leaves 1/2 cup Parmigiano-Reggiano cheese, preferably freshly grated 1/2 cup olive oil

Directions

Place the chicken legs in a parchnemt-lined baking pan. Season with salt and pepper, Then, scatter the leeks around the chicken legs. Roast in the preheated oven at 390 degrees F for 30 to 35 minutes, rotating the pan occasionally. Pulse the cashews, basil, garlic, and cheese in your blender until pieces are small. Continue blending while adding olive oil to the mixture. Mix until the desired consistency is reached.Bon appétit!

63. Turkey Chorizo with Bok Choy

(Ready in about 50 minutes | Servings 4) Per serving: 189 Calories; 12g Fat; 2.6g Carbs; 9.4g Protein; 1g Fiber

Ingredients

4 mild turkey Chorizo, sliced 1/2 cup full-fat milk 6 ounces Gruyère cheese, preferably freshly grated 1 yellow onion, chopped Coarse salt and ground black pepper, to taste 1 pound Bok choy, tough stem ends trimmed 1 cup cream of mushroom soup 1 tablespoon lard, room temperature

Directions

Melt the lard in a nonstick skillet over a moderate flame; cook the Chorizo sausage for about 5 minutes, stirring occasionally to ensure even cooking; reserve. Add in the onion, salt, pepper, Bok choy, and cream of mushroom soup. Continue to cook for 4 minutes longer or until the vegetables have softened. Spoon the mixture into a lightly oiled casserole dish. Top with the reserved Chorizo. In a mixing bowl, thoroughly combine the milk and cheese. Pour the cheese mixture over the sausage. Cover with foil and bake at 365 degrees F for about 35 minutes.Enjoy!

64. Taro Leaf and Chicken Soup

(Ready in about 45 minutes | Servings 4) Per serving: 256 Calories; 12.9g Fat; 3.2g Carbs; 35.1g Protein; 2.2g Fiber

Ingredients

1 pound whole chicken, boneless and chopped into small chunks 1/2 cup onions, chopped 1/2 cup rutabaga, cubed 2 carrots, peeled 2 celery stalks Salt and black pepper, to taste 1 cup chicken bone broth 1/2 teaspoon ginger-garlic paste 1/2 cup taro leaves, roughly chopped 1 tablespoon fresh coriander, chopped 3 cups water 1 teaspoon paprika

Directions Place all ingredients in a heavy-bottomed pot. Bring to a boil over the highest heat. Turn the heat to simmer. Continue to cook, partially covered, an additional 40 minutes. Storing Spoon the soup into four airtight containers or Ziploc bags; keep in your refrigerator for up to 3 to 4 days. For freezing, place the soup in airtight containers. It will maintain the best quality for about 5 to 6 months. Defrost in the refrigerator. Bon appétit!

65. Italian-Style Chicken Meatballs with Parmesan

(Ready in about 20 minutes | Servings 6) Per serving: 252 Calories; 9.7g Fat; 5.3g Carbs; 34.2g Protein; 1.4g Fiber

Ingredients

For the Meatballs: 1 ¼ pounds chicken, ground 1 tablespoon sage leaves, chopped 1 teaspoon shallot powder 1 teaspoon porcini powder 2 garlic cloves, finely minced 1/3 teaspoon dried basil 3/4 cup Parmesan cheese, grated 2 eggs, lightly beaten Salt and ground black pepper, to your liking 1/2 teaspoon cayenne pepper For the sauce: 2 tomatoes, pureed 1 cup chicken consommé 2 ½ tablespoons lard, room temperature 1 onion, peeled and finely chopped

Directions In a mixing bowl, combine all ingredients for the meatballs. Roll the mixture into bite-sized balls. Melt 1 tablespoon of lard in a skillet over a moderately high heat. Sear the meatballs for about 3 minutes or until they are thoroughly cooked; reserve. Melt the remaining lard and cook the onions until tender and translucent. Add in pureed tomatoes and chicken consommé and continue to cook for 4 minutes longer. Add in the reserved meatballs, turn the heat to simmer and continue to cook for 6 to 7 minutes. Bon appétit!

66. Spicy Chicken Breasts

(Ready in about 30 minutes | Servings 6) Per serving: 239 Calories; 8.6g Fat; 5.5g Carbs; 34.3g Protein; 1g Fiber

Ingredients

1 ½ pounds chicken breasts 1 bell pepper, deveined and chopped 1 leek, chopped 1 tomato, pureed 2 tablespoons coriander 2 garlic cloves, minced 1 teaspoon cayenne pepper 1 teaspoon dry thyme 1/4 cup coconut aminos Sea salt and ground black pepper, to taste

Directions

Rub each chicken breasts with the garlic, cayenne pepper, thyme, salt and black pepper. Cook the chicken in a saucepan over medium-high heat. Sear for about 5 minutes until golden brown on all sides. Fold in the tomato puree and coconut aminos and bring it to a boil. Add in the pepper, leek, and coriander. Reduce the heat to simmer. Continue to cook, partially covered, for about 20 minutes.Bon appétit!

67. Spicy and Cheesy Turkey Dip

(Ready in about 25 minutes | Servings 4) Per serving: 284 Calories; 19g Fat; 3.2g Carbs; 26.7g Protein; 1.6g Fiber

Ingredients

1 Fresno chili pepper, deveined and minced 1 ½ cups Ricotta cheese, creamed, 4% fat, softened 1/4 cup sour cream 1 tablespoon butter, room temperature 1 shallot, chopped 1 teaspoon garlic, pressed 1 pound ground turkey 1/2 cup goat cheese, shredded Salt and black pepper, to taste 1 ½ cups Gruyère, shredded

Directions

Melt the butter in a frying pan over a moderately high flame. Now, sauté the onion and garlic until they have softened. Stir in the ground turkey and continue to cook until it is no longer pink. Transfer the sautéed mixture to a lightly greased baking dish. Add in Ricotta, sour cream, goat cheese, salt, pepper, and chili pepper. Top with the shredded Gruyère cheese. Bake in the preheated oven at 350 degrees F for about 20 minutes or until hot and bubbly in top.Enjoy!

68. Spicy and Tangy Chicken Drumsticks

(Ready in about 55 minutes | Servings 6) Per serving: 420 Calories; 28.2g Fat; 5g Carbs; 35.3g Protein; 0.8g Fiber

Ingredients

3 chicken drumsticks, cut into chunks 1/2 stick butter 2 eggs 1/4 cup hemp seeds, ground Salt and cayenne pepper, to taste 2 tablespoons coconut aminos 3 teaspoons red wine vinegar 2 tablespoons salsa 2 cloves garlic, minced

Directions

Rub the chicken with the butter, salt, and cayenne pepper. Drizzle the chicken with the coconut aminos, vinegar, salsa, and garlic. Allow it to stand for 30 minutes in your refrigerator. Whisk the eggs with the hemp seeds. Dip each chicken strip in the egg mixture. Place the chicken chunks in a parchment-lined baking pan. Roast in the preheated oven at 390 degrees F for 25 minutes.Enjoy!

69. Mexican-Style Turkey Bacon Bites

(Ready in about 5 minutes | Servings 4) Per serving: 195 Calories; 16.7g Fat; 2.2g Carbs; 8.8g Protein; 0.3g Fiber

Ingredients

4 ounces turkey bacon, chopped 4 ounces Neufchatel cheese 1 tablespoon butter, cold 1 jalapeno pepper, deveined and minced 1 teaspoon Mexican oregano 2 tablespoons . scallions, finely chopped

Directions

Thoroughly combine all ingredients in a mixing bowl. Roll the mixture into 8 balls.

70. Bacon-Wrapped Chicken with Grilled Asparagus

Ready in about: 50 minutes | Serves: 4 Per serving: Kcal 468, Fat 38g, Net Carbs 2g, Protein 26g

Ingredients

4 chicken breasts Pink salt and black pepper to taste 8 bacon slices 2 tbsp olive oil 1 lb asparagus spears 3 tbsp olive oil 2 tbsp fresh lemon juice 2 oz Manchego cheese for topping Preheat oven to 400°F.

DirectionsSeason the chicken breasts with salt and pepper. Wrap 2 bacon slices around each chicken breast. Arrange them on a baking sheet, drizzle with olive oil, and bake for 25-30 minutes until the bacon is brown and crispy. Remove and cover with foil to keep warm. Preheat grill to high heat. Brush the asparagus with olive oil and season with salt. Grill for 8-10 minutes, frequently turning until slightly charred. Remove to a plate and drizzle with lemon juice. Grate over Manchego cheese to melts a little on contact with the hot asparagus and forms a cheesy dressing. Serve.

71. Chicken Drumsticks in Tomato Sauce

Ready in about: 1 ½ hours | Serves: 4 Per serving: Kcal 515, Fat 34.2g, Net Carbs 7.3g, Protein 50.8g

Ingredients

8 chicken drumsticks 2 tbsp olive oil 1 medium white onion, chopped 2 medium turnips, peeled and diced 1 medium carrot, chopped 2 green bell peppers, cut into chunks 2 cloves garlic, minced ¼ cup coconut flour 1 cup chicken broth 1 (28 oz) can sugar-free tomato sauce 2 tbsp dried Italian herbs Salt and black pepper to taste Preheat oven to 400°F.

DirectionsHeat the olive oil in a skillet over medium heat. Season the drumsticks with salt and pepper and fry for 10 minutes on all sides until brown. Remove to a baking dish. Sauté the onion, turnips, bell peppers, carrot, and garlic in the same oil for 10 minutes with continuous stirring. In a bowl, combine the broth, coconut flour, tomato paste, and Italian herbs together and pour it over the vegetables in the skillet. Stir and cook for 4 minutes until thickened. Pour the mixture over the chicken in the baking dish. Bake for around 1 hour. Remove from the oven and serve with steamed cauli rice.

72. Sweet Garlic Chicken Skewers

Ready in about: 20 minutes + time refrigeration | Serves: 4 Per serving: Kcal 225, Fat 17.4g, Net Carbs 2g, Protein 15g

Ingredients

Skewers 3 tbsp soy sauce 1 tbsp ginger-garlic paste 2 tbsp swerve brown sugar 1 tsp chili pepper 2 tbsp olive oil 1 lb chicken breasts, cut into cubes Dressing ½ cup tahini ½ tsp garlic powder Pink salt to taste

Directions

In a bowl, whisk soy sauce, ginger-garlic paste, swerve brown sugar, chili pepper, and olive oil. Put the chicken in a zipper bag. Pour in the marinade, seal, and shake to coat. Marinate in the fridge for 2 hours. Preheat grill to 400°F. Thread the chicken on skewers. Cook for 10 minutes in total with three to four turnings until golden brown; remove to a plate. Mix the tahini, garlic powder, salt, and ¼ cup of warm water in a bowl. Pour into serving jars. Serve the chicken skewers and tahini dressing with cauli rice.

73. Parmesan Wings with Yogurt

Sauce Ready in about: 25 minutes | Serves: 6 Per serving: Kcal 452, Fat 36.4g, Net Carbs 4g, Protein 24g

Ingredients

1 cup Greek-style yogurt 2 tbsp extra-virgin olive oil 1 tbsp fresh dill, chopped 2 lb chicken wings Salt and black pepper to taste ½ cup butter, melted ½ cup hot sauce ¼ cup Parmesan cheese, grated Preheat oven to 400°F.

Directions

Mix yogurt, olive oil, dill, salt, and black pepper in a bowl. Chill while making the chicken. Season wings with salt and pepper. Line them on a baking sheet and grease with cooking spray. Bake for 20 minutes until golden brown. Mix butter, hot sauce, and Parmesan cheese in a bowl. Toss chicken in the sauce to evenly coat and plate. Serve with yogurt dipping sauce.

74. Chicken Cauliflower Bake

Ready in about: 50 minutes | Serves: 6 Per serving: Kcal 390, Fat 27g, Net Carbs 3g, Protein 22g

Ingredients

3 cups cubed leftover chicken 3 cups spinach 2 cauliflower heads, cut into florets 3 eggs, lightly beaten 2 cups grated sharp cheddar cheese 1 cup pork rinds, crushed ½ cup unsweetened almond milk 3 tbsp olive oil 3 cloves garlic, minced Preheat oven to 350°F.

DirectionsPour the cauli florets and 3 cups water in a pot over medium heat and bring to a boil. Cover and steam the cauli florets for 8 minutes. Drain through a colander and set aside. Combine the cheddar cheese and pork rinds in a large bowl and mix in the chicken. Set aside. Heat the olive oil in a skillet and cook the garlic and spinach until the spinach has wilted, about 5 minutes. Add the spinach mixture and cauli florets to the chicken bowl. Add in the eggs and almond milk, mix, and transfer everything to a greased baking dish. Layer the top of the ingredients. Place the dish in the oven and bake for 30 minutes. By this time, the edges and top must have browned nicely. Remove the chicken from the oven, let rest for 5 minutes, and serve.

75. Easy Chicken Chili

Ready in about: 30 minutes | Serves: 4 Per serving: Kcal: 421, Fat: 21g, Net Carbs: 5.6g, Protein: 45g

Ingredients 4 chicken breasts 2 tbsp butter 1 onion, chopped 8 oz diced tomatoes 2 tbsp tomato puree ½ tsp chili powder ½ tsp cumin ½ tsp garlic powder 1 serrano pepper, minced ½ cup cheddar cheese, shredded Salt and black pepper to taste

Directions Put a large saucepan over medium heat and add the chicken. Cover with water and bring to a boil. Cook for 10 minutes. Transfer the chicken to a flat surface and shred with forks. Reserve 2 cups of the broth. Melt the butter in a large pot over medium heat. Sauté onion until transparent for 3 minutes. Stir in the chicken, tomatoes, cumin, serrano pepper, garlic powder, tomato puree, broth, and chili powder. Adjust the seasoning and let the mixture boil. Simmer for 10 minutes. Top with shredded cheese and serve.

76. Lemon-Garlic Chicken Skewers

Ready in about: 20 minutes + marinating time | Serves: 4 Per serving: Kcal 350, Fat 11g, Net Carbs 3.5g, Protein 34g

Ingredients 1 lb chicken breasts, cut into cubes 2 tbsp olive oil 2/3 jar preserved lemon, drained 2 garlic cloves, minced ½ cup lemon juice Salt and black pepper to taste 1 tsp fresh rosemary, chopped 4 lemon wedges

Directions In a wide bowl, mix half of the oil, garlic, salt, pepper, and lemon juice and add the chicken cubes and lemon rind. Let marinate for 2 hours in the refrigerator. Remove the chicken and thread it onto skewers. Heat a grill pan over high heat. Add in the chicken skewers and sear them for 6 minutes per side. Remove to a plate and serve warm garnished with rosemary and lemons wedges.

77. Cheese & Spinach Stuffed Chicken Breasts

Ready in about: 50 minutes | Serves: 4 Per serving: Kcal 491, Fat: 36g, Net Carbs: 3.5g, Protein: 38g

Ingredients 4 chicken breasts ½ cup mozzarella cheese, grated ⅓ cup Parmesan cheese 6 oz cream cheese, softened 2 cups spinach, chopped ½ tsp ground nutmeg Breading 2 eggs ⅓ cup almond flour 2 tbsp olive oil ½ tsp parsley ⅓ cup Parmesan cheese 1 tsp onion powder

Directions Pound the chicken until it doubles in size. Mix the cream cheese, spinach, mozzarella cheese, nutmeg, salt, black pepper, and Parmesan cheese in a bowl. Divide the mixture between the chicken breasts. Close the chicken around the filling. Wrap the breasts with cling film. Refrigerate for 15 minutes. Preheat oven to 370°F. Beat the eggs in a shallow dish. Combine all other breading ingredients in a bowl. Dip the chicken in egg first, then in the breading mixture. Heat the olive oil in a pan over medium heat. Cook chicken for 3-5 minutes on all sides. Transfer to a baking sheet. Bake for 20 minutes. Serve.

78. Greek Chicken with Capers

Ready in about: 30 minutes | Serves: 4 Per serving: Kcal 387, Fat 21g, Net Carbs 2.2g, Protein 25g

Ingredients

½ cup Kalamata olives, pitted and chopped ¼ cup olive oil 1 onion, chopped 4 chicken breasts 2 garlic cloves, minced Salt and black pepper to taste 1 tbsp capers 1 lb tomatoes, chopped ½ tsp red chili flakes

DirectionsSprinkle black pepper and salt on the chicken and brush with some olive oil. Add it to a pan set over high heat and cook for 2 minutes. Flip to the other side and cook for 2 more minutes. Transfer the chicken breasts to the oven and bake for 8 minutes at 450°F. Split the chicken into serving plates. Put the same pan over medium heat and warm the remaining oil. Place in the onion, olives, capers, garlic, and chili flakes and cook for 1 minute. Stir in the tomatoes, black pepper, and salt, and cook for 2 minutes. Sprinkle over the chicken breasts and serve.

79. Chicken in Creamy Tomato Sauce

Ready in about: 25 minutes | Serves: 6 Per serving: Kcal 456, Fat 38.2g, Net Carbs 2g, Protein 24g

Ingredients

3 tbsp butter 6 chicken thighs Salt and black pepper to taste 14 oz canned tomato sauce 2 tsp Italian seasoning ½ cup heavy cream 1 cup mozzarella cheese, shredded ½ cup Parmesan cheese, grated

DirectionsIn a saucepan, melt the butter over medium heat. Season the chicken with salt and black pepper and brown for 5 minutes on each side. Plate the chicken. Pour the tomato sauce and Italian seasoning in the pan and cook for 8 minutes. Adjust the taste with salt and black pepper. Stir in the heavy cream and mozzarella cheese. Once the cheese has melted, return the chicken to the pot and simmer for 4 minutes. Remove to a plate, garnish with Parmesan cheese, and serve.

80. Spicy Chicken Kebabs

Ready in about: 20 minutes + marinade time | Serves: 6 Per serving: Kcal 198, Fat: 13.5g, Net Carbs: 3.1g, Protein: 17.5g

Ingredients

2 lb chicken breasts, cubed 3 tbsp sesame oil 1 cup red bell peppers, chopped 2 tbsp five-spice powder 2 tbsp granulated sweetener 1 tbsp fish sauce

DirectionsCombine the sesame oil, fish sauce, five-spice powder, and granulated sweetener in a bowl and mix well. Add in the chicken and toss to coat. Let marinate for 1 hour in the fridge. Preheat the grill. Thread the chicken and bell peppers onto skewers. Grill for 3 minutes per side. Serve warm with steamed broccoli.

81. Roasted Chicken Kabobs with Celery Fries

Ready in about: 50 minutes | Serves: 4 Per serving: Kcal: 579, Fat: 43g, Net Carbs: 6g, Protein: 39g

Ingredients

1 lb chicken breasts, cubed 4 tbsp olive oil 1 cup chicken broth 1 head celery root, sliced 2 tbsp olive oil Salt and black pepper to taste Preheat oven to 400°F.

Directions

In a bowl, mix 2 tbsp of the olive oil, salt, and pepper. Add in the chicken and toss to coat. Cover with foil and place in the fridge. Arrange the celery slices in a baking tray in an even layer and coat with the remaining olive oil. Season with salt and black pepper and place in the oven. Bake for 10 minutes. Take out the chicken of the refrigerator and thread it onto skewers. Place over the celery, pour in the chicken broth, and roast in the oven for 30 minutes. Serve warm in plates.

82. Chicken Garam Masala

Ready in about: 35 minutes | Serves: 4 Per serving: Kcal: 564, Fat: 50g, Net Carbs: 5g, Protein: 33g

Ingredients

1 lb chicken breasts, cut lengthwise 2 tbsp butter 1 tbsp olive oil 1 yellow bell pepper, finely chopped 1 ¼ cups heavy whipping cream 1 tbsp fresh cilantro, finely chopped Salt and pepper, to taste Garam masala 1 tsp ground cumin 2 tsp ground coriander 1 tsp ground cardamom 1 tsp turmeric 1 tsp ginger 1 tsp paprika 1 tsp cayenne, ground 1 pinch ground nutmeg Preheat oven to 400°F.

DirectionsIn a bowl, mix the garam masala spices. Coat the chicken with half of the mixture. Heat the olive oil and butter in a frying pan over medium heat. Brown the chicken for 3 minutes per side. Transfer to a baking dish. To the remaining masala, add heavy cream, bell pepper, salt, and pepper. Pour over the chicken. Bake for 20 minutes until the mixture starts to bubble. Garnish with cilantro to serve.

83. Yummy Chicken Nuggets

Ready in about: 25 minutes | Serves: 2 Per serving: Kcal 417, Fat 37g, Net Carbs 4.3g, Protein 35g

Ingredients ½ cup almond flour 1 egg, beaten ½ tsp garlic powder 2 chicken breasts, cut into chunks Salt and black pepper to taste ½ cup butter

DirectionsIn a bowl, mix salt, garlic powder, flour, and pepper and stir. Dip the chicken chunks in egg, then in the flour mixture. Warm butter in a pan over medium heat. Add in the chicken nuggets and cook for 6 minutes on each side. Remove to paper towels, drain the excess grease, and serve with your favorite dip.

84. Stuffed Avocados with Chicken

Ready in about: 10 minutes | Serves: 2 Per serving: Kcal 511, Fat 40, Net Carbs 5g, Protein 24g

Ingredients

2 avocados, cut in half and pitted ¼ cup pesto 2 tbsp cream cheese 1 ½ cups chicken, cooked, shredded ¼ tsp cayenne pepper ½ tsp onion powder ½ tsp garlic powder Salt and black pepper to taste 2 tbsp lemon juice

Directions

Scoop the insides of the avocado halves, and place the flesh in a bowl. Add in the chicken and stir in the remaining ingredients. Stuff the avocado cups with chicken mixture and enjoy.

85. Homemade Chicken Pizza Calzone

Ready in about: 60 minutes | Serves: 4 Per serving: Kcal 425, Fat 15g, Net Carbs 4.6g, Protein 28g

Ingredients

2 eggs 1 low carb pizza crust ½ cup Pecorino cheese, grated ½ lb chicken breasts, halved ½ cup sugar-free marinara sauce 1 tsp Italian seasoning 1 tsp onion powder Salt and black pepper to taste ¼ cup flax seed, ground 1 cup provolone cheese, grated

Directions

In a bowl, combine the Italian seasoning with onion powder, salt, Pecorino cheese, pepper, and flaxseed. In a separate bowl, beat the eggs with pepper and salt. Dip the chicken pieces in eggs and then in cheese mixture. Lay them on a lined baking sheet and bake for 25 minutes in the oven at 390°F. Remove the chicken from the oven and leave it to cool slightly before chopping. Place the pizza dough on a lined baking sheet. Spread ½ cup of the provolone cheese on 1 half of the crust, leaving a ⅓ inch edge around the trim. Scatter the chopped chicken over the cheese and top with marinara sauce. Sprinkle with the remaining cheese. Fold the other half of the dough over the filling. Seal the edges, set in the oven, and bake for 20 minutes. Allow the calzone to cool down before slicing. Serve.

86. Easy Chicken Meatloaf

Ready in about: 50 minutes | Serves: 6 Per serving: Kcal 273, Fat 14g, Net Carbs 4g, Protein 28

Ingredients

1 cup sugar-free marinara sauce 2 lb ground chicken 2 garlic cloves, minced 2 tsp onion powder 1 tsp Italian seasoning Salt and black pepper to taste Filling ½ cup ricotta cheese 1 cup Grana Padano cheese, grated 1 cup Colby cheese, shredded 2 tsp fresh chives, chopped 2 tbsp fresh parsley, chopped

Directions

In a bowl, combine the ground chicken with half of the marinara sauce, pepper, onion powder, Italian seasoning, salt, and garlic. In a separate bowl, mix the ricotta cheese with half of the Grana Padano cheese, chives, pepper, half of the Colby cheese, salt, and parsley. Place half of the chicken mixture into a loaf pan and spread evenly. Top with the cheese filling. Cover with the rest of the chicken mixture and spread again. Set the meatloaf in the preheated to 380°F oven. Bake for 25 minutes. Remove meatloaf and spread the rest of the marinara sauce, Grana Padano cheese, and Colby cheese. Bake for 18 minutes. Allow meatloaf cooling and serve in sliced.

87. Thyme Chicken Thighs

Ready in about: 30 minutes | Serves: 4 Per serving: Kcal 528, Fat: 42g, Net Carbs: 4g, Protein: 33g

Ingredients

½ cup chicken stock 2 tbsp olive oil 1 onion, chopped 4 chicken thighs ¼ cup heavy cream 2 tbsp Dijon mustard 1 tsp thyme 1 tsp garlic powder

Directions

Heat the olive oil in a pan over medium heat. Cook the chicken for about 4 minutes per side. Set aside. Sauté the onion in the same pan for 3 minutes, add the stock, and simmer for 5 minutes. Stir in mustard, heavy cream, thyme, and garlic powder. Pour the sauce over the chicken and serve.

88. Grilled Paprika Chicken with Steamed Broccoli

Ready in about: 17 minutes | Serves: 6 Per serving: Kcal 422, Fat 35.3g, Net Carbs 2g, Protein 26g

Ingredients

1 tsp smoked paprika Salt and black pepper to taste 1 tsp garlic powder 3 tbsp olive oil 6 chicken breasts 1 head broccoli, cut into florets

Directions

Place broccoli florets onto the steamer basket over the boiling water and steam for 8 minutes or until crisp-tender. Set aside. Preheat grill to high and grease the grate with cooking spray Mix paprika, salt, pepper, and garlic powder in a bowl. Brush chicken with olive oil, sprinkle spice mixture over, and massage with hands. Grill chicken for 7 minutes per side until well-cooked. Serve warm.

89. Chicken Goujons with Tomato Sauce

Ready in about: 50 minutes | Serves: 6 Per serving: Kcal 415, Fat 36g, Net Carbs 5g, Protein 28g

Ingredients 1 ½ lb chicken breasts, cubed Salt and black pepper to taste 1 egg, beaten in a bowl 1 cup almond flour ¼ cup Parmesan cheese, grated ½ tsp garlic powder ½ tsp dried parsley ½ tsp dried basil 4 tbsp avocado oil 4 cups butternut squash spirals 6 oz Gruyere cheese, shredded 1½ cups tomato sauce

Directions In a bowl, combine the almond flour, Parmesan cheese, pepper, and garlic powder. Dip the chicken in the egg first, and then in the almond flour mixture. Set a pan over medium heat and warm 3 tablespoons avocado oil. Add in the chicken and cook until golden, about 5-6 minutes. Remove to paper towels. In a bowl, combine the butternut squash spirals with salt, dried basil, remaining avocado oil, and black pepper. Transfer to a baking dish and top with the chicken pieces, followed by the tomato sauce. Scatter shredded Gruyere cheese on top and bake for 30 minutes at 360ºF. Remove and serve.

90. Chicken with Anchovy Tapenade

Ready in about: 30 minutes | Serves: 2 Per serving: Kcal 155, Fat 13g, Net Carbs 3g, Protein 25g

Ingredients 1 chicken breast, cut into 4 pieces 1 tbsp coconut oil 2 garlic cloves, crushed Anchovy tapenade ½ cup black olives, pitted 1 oz anchovy fillets, rinsed 1 garlic clove, crushed Salt and black pepper to taste 1 tbsp olive oil 1 tbsp lemon juice

Directions Blend the tapenade ingredients in a food processor until smooth and set aside. Warm the coconut oil in a pan over medium heat. Stir in the garlic and sauté for 1 minute. Add in the chicken pieces and cook each side for 4 minutes. Top the chicken with the anchovy tapenade and serve.

91. Baked Chicken with Parmesan Topping

Ready in about: 45 minutes | Serves: 4 Per serving: Kcal 361, Fat 15g, Net Carbs 5g, Protein 25g

Ingredients

4 chicken breast halves Salt and black pepper to taste ¼ cup green chilies, chopped 4 bacon slices, chopped 4 oz cream cheese, softened 1 onion, chopped ½ cup mayonnaise ½ cup Grana Padano cheese, grated 1 cup cheddar cheese, grated 2 oz pork rinds, crushed 2 tbsp olive oil ½ cup Parmesan cheese, shredded Season the chicken with salt and pepper.

Directions

Heat the olive oil in a pan over medium heat and fry the chicken for about 4-6 minutes until cooked through with no pink showing. Remove to a baking dish. In the same pan, fry bacon until crispy and remove to a plate. Sauté the onion in the same fat for 3 minutes until soft. Remove from heat, add in the fried bacon, cream cheese, 1 cup of water, Grana Padano cheese, mayonnaise, chilies, and cheddar cheese and spread over the chicken. Bake in the oven for 10-15 minutes at 370°F. Remove and sprinkle with mixed Parmesan cheese and pork rinds and return to the oven. Bake for another 10-15 minutes until the cheese melts. Serve immediately.

---

92. Cheddar Chicken Tenders

Ready in about: 35 minutes | Serves: 4 Per serving: Kcal 507, Fat 54g, Net Carbs 1.3g, Protein 42g

Ingredients

2 eggs 2 tbsp butter, melted 3 cups cheddar cheese, crushed ½ cup pork rinds, crushed 1 lb chicken tenders Pink salt to taste Preheat oven to 350°F. Line a baking sheet with parchment paper.

Directions

Whisk the eggs with butter in a bowl. Mix the cheese and pork rinds in another bowl. Season the chicken with salt. Dip it in the egg mixture. Coat with the cheddar mixture. Place on the baking sheet, cover with aluminium foil, and bake for 15 minutes. Remove foil and bake for 10 more minutes until golden brown. Serve chicken with mustard dip.

93. Bacon & Cheese Chicken

Ready in about: 30 minutes | Serves: 4 Per serving: Kcal 423, Fat 21g, Net Carbs 3.3g, Protein 34g

Ingredients

4 bacon strips 4 chicken breasts 2 tbsp avocado jalapeño sauce 1 oz coconut aminos 2 tbsp coconut oil 4 oz Monterey Jack cheese, grated

DirectionsHeat a pan over medium heat and add in the bacon. Cook for 5 minutes until crispy. Remove to paper towels, drain the grease, and crumble. To the pan, add and warm the coconut oil. Place in the chicken breasts, cook for 4 minutes, flip, and cook for an additional 4 minutes. Transfer to a baking dish. Top with the coconut aminos, Monterey Jack cheese, and crumbled bacon. Insert in the oven, turn on the broiler, and cook for 5 minutes. Serve topped with avocado jalapeño sauce.

94. Chicken with Tarragon

Ready in about: 50 minutes | Serves: 4 Per serving: Kcal: 415, Fat: 23g, Net Carbs: 5.5g, Protein: 42g

Ingredients

1 lb chicken thighs 1 lb radishes, sliced 2 oz butter, sliced 1 tbsp tarragon Salt and black pepper to taste 1 cup mayonnaise Preheat oven to 400°F.

Directions

Place the chicken on a greased baking dish. Add in radishes and season with tarragon, pepper, and salt. Top with butter and bake in the oven for 40 minutes. Serve with mayonnaise.

95. Pacific Chicken

Ready in about: 50 minutes | Serves: 6 Per serving: Kcal: 465, Fat: 31g, Net Carbs: 2.6g, Protein: 33g

Ingredients 4 chicken breasts Salt and black pepper to taste ½ cup mayonnaise 1 tbsp Dijon mustard 1 tsp xylitol ¾ cup pork rinds, crushed ¾ cup Grana Padano cheese, grated 1 tsp garlic powder 1 tsp onion powder Salt and black pepper to taste 8 pieces ham, sliced 4 Gruyere cheese slices

DirectionsPreheat oven to 350°F. In a bowl, mix mustard, mayonnaise, and xylitol. Rub the mixture onto the chicken. In another bowl, combine the pork rinds, garlic and onion powders, salt, pepper, and Grana Padano cheese. Pour half of the mixture in a greased baking dish. Add the chicken to the top. Cover with the remaining pork rind mixture. Roast for 40 minutes until the chicken is cooked thoroughly. Take out from the oven and top with Gruyere cheese and ham. Place back in the oven and cook until golden brown. Serve warm.

96. Coconut Chicken Soup

Ready in about: 30 minutes | Serves: 4 Per serving: Kcal 387, Fat 23g, Net Carbs 5g, Protein 31g

Ingredients

2 tbsp coconut oil 1-inch piece peeled ginger, grated 2 chicken breasts, diced 4 cups chicken stock ½ cup coconut cream ¼ cup celery, chopped 1 cup mushrooms, sliced 1 tbsp lime juice ½ tsp red pepper flakes 2 tbsp fresh cilantro, chopped 2 tbsp fish sauce Salt and black pepper to taste

Directions

Warm the coconut oil in a large saucepan over medium heat. Add in the chicken, ginger, mushrooms, and celery and sauté for 3-4 minutes, stirring occasionally. Pour in the chicken stock, fish sauce, lime juice, and pepper flakes and bring to a boil. Reduce the heat and simmer for 18-20 minutes. Whisk in the coconut cream and season with salt and pepper. Continue cooking for about 5 minutes. Garnish with cilantro, spoon onto soup bowls, and serve.

97. Slow Cooker Chicken Stroganoff

Ready in about: 4 hours 15 minutes | Serves: 4 Per serving: Kcal 365, Fat 22g, Net Carbs 4g, Protein 26g

Ingredients

2 garlic cloves, minced 8 oz mushrooms, chopped ¼ tsp celery seeds, ground 1 cup chicken stock 1 cup sour cream 1 cup leeks, chopped 1 lb chicken breasts ½ tsp dried thyme 2 tbsp fresh parsley, chopped Salt and black pepper to taste 4 zucchinis, spiralized 2 tbsp olive oil

Directions

Place the chicken in the slow cooker. Season with salt and pepper and add in the leeks, sour cream, parsley, celery seeds, garlic, mushrooms, stock, and thyme. Cover and cook on high for 4 hours on High. Heat the olive oil in a pan over medium heat. Add in the zucchini pasta and cook for 1-2 minutes until tender. Divide the zucchini between serving plates, top with the chicken mixture, and serve.

98. One-Pot Chicken with Mushrooms & Spinach

Ready in about: 40 minutes | Serves: 4 Per serving: Kcal 453, Fat 23g, Net Carbs 1g, Protein 32g

Ingredients

1 lb chicken thighs 1 cup mushrooms, sliced 2 cups spinach, chopped ¼ cup butter Salt and black pepper to taste ½ tsp onion powder ½ tsp garlic powder 1 tsp Dijon mustard 1 tbsp fresh tarragon, chopped

Directions

Melt the butter in a pan over medium heat. Add in the thighs, onion powder, pepper, garlic powder, and salt. Cook each side for 3 minutes. Set aside. To the same pan, add the mushrooms and cook for 5 minutes. Place in ½ cup water and mustard, take the chicken pieces back to the pan, and cook for 15 minutes while covered. Stir in the tarragon and spinach and cook for 5 minutes. Serve warm.

99. Stuffed Mushrooms with Chicken

Ready in about: 40 minutes | Serves: 4 Per serving: Kcal 261, Fat 16g, Net Carbs 6g, Protein 14g

Ingredients 8 portobello mushrooms, stems removed 3 cups cauliflower florets Salt and black pepper to taste 1 onion, chopped 1 lb ground chicken 2 tbsp butter ½ cup vegetable broth

Direction In a food processor, add the cauliflower florets, pepper, and salt and blend until it has a rice texture. Transfer to a plate. Warm the butter in a pan over medium heat. Stir in onion and cook for 3 minutes. Add in the cauliflower rice and ground chicken and cook for 5 minutes. Stir in the broth, salt, and pepper and cook for further 2 minutes. Arrange the mushrooms on a lined baking sheet, stuff each one with chicken mixture, put in the oven, and bake for 30 minutes at 350°F. Place on serving plates and enjoy!

100.   Paprika Chicken with Cream Sauce

Ready in about: 50 minutes | Serves: 4 Per serving: Kcal 381, Fat 33g, Net Carbs 2.6g, Protein 31.3g

Ingredients

1 lb chicken thighs Salt and black pepper to taste 1 tsp onion powder ¼ cup heavy cream 2 tbsp butter 2 tbsp sweet paprika In a bowl, combine paprika with onion powder, pepper, and salt.

Directions Rub the chicken with the mixture and lay on a lined baking sheet. Bake for 40 minutes in the oven at 400°F. Set aside. Add the cooking juices to a skillet over medium heat, and mix with the heavy cream and butter. Cook for 5-6 minutes until the sauce is thickened. Sprinkle the sauce over the chicken and serve.

101. Chicken Breasts with Spinach & Artichoke

Ready in about: 40 minutes | Serves: 4 Per serving: Kcal 431, Fat 21g, Net Carbs 3.5g, Protein 36g

Ingredients

4 oz cream cheese, softened 4 chicken breasts 8 oz canned artichoke hearts 1 cup spinach ½ cup Pecorino cheese, grated ½ tsp onion powder ½ tbsp garlic powder Salt and black pepper to taste 4 oz Monterrey Jack cheese, grated

Directions

Lay the chicken breasts on a lined baking sheet, season with pepper and salt, and set in the preheated oven at 350°F. Bake for 25 minutes. Chop the artichoke hearts and place them in a bowl. Add in onion powder, Pecorino cheese, salt, spinach, cream cheese, garlic powder, and pepper and toss to combine. Remove the chicken from the oven and cut each piece in half lengthwise. Divide the artichokes mixture on top, sprinkle with Monterrey cheese, and return in the oven. Bake for 10 minutes. Serve warm.

102. Country-Style Chicken Stew

(Ready in about 1 hour | Servings 6) Per serving: 280 Calories; 14.7g Fat; 2.5g Carbs; 25.6g Protein; 2.5g Fiber

Ingredients

1 pound chicken thighs 2 tablespoons butter, room temperature 1/2 pound carrots, chopped 1 bell pepper, chopped 1 chile pepper, deveined and minced 1 cup tomato puree Kosher salt and ground black pepper, to taste 1/2 teaspoon smoked paprika 1 onion, finely chopped 1 teaspoon garlic, sliced 4 cups vegetable broth 1 teaspoon dried basil 1 celery, chopped

Directions

Melt the butter in a stockpot over medium-high flame. Sweat the onion and garlic until just tender and fragrant. Reduce the heat to medium-low. Stir in the broth, chicken thighs, and basil; bring to a rolling boil. Add in the remaining ingredients. Partially cover and let it simmer for 45 to 50 minutes. Shred the meat, discarding the bones; add the chicken back to the pot.Bon appétit!

103. Panna Cotta with Chicken and Bleu d' Auvergne

(Ready in about 20 minutes + chilling time | Servings 4) Per serving: 306 Calories; 18.3g Fat; 4.7g Carbs; 29.5g Protein; 0g Fiber

Ingredients

2 chicken legs, boneless and skinless 1 tablespoon avocado oil 2 teaspoons granular erythritol 3 tablespoons water 1 cup Bleu d' Auvergne, crumbled 2 gelatin sheets 3/4 cup double cream Salt and cayenne pepper, to your liking

Directions

Heat the oil in a frying pan over medium-high heat; fry the chicken for about 10 minutes. Soak the gelatin sheets in cold water. Cook with the cream, erythritol, water, and Bleu d' Auvergne. Season with salt and pepper and let it simmer over the low heat, stirring for about 3 minutes. Spoon the mixture into four ramekins.Enjoy!

104. Chicken Drumsticks with Broccoli and Cheese

(Ready in about 1 hour 15 minutes | Servings 4) Per serving: 533 Calories; 40.2g Fat; 5.4g Carbs; 35.1g Protein; 3.5g Fiber

Ingredients

1 pound chicken drumsticks 1 pound broccoli, broken into florets 2 cups cheddar cheese, shredded 1/2 teaspoon dried oregano 1/2 teaspoon dried basil 3 tablespoons olive oil 1 celery, sliced 1 cup green onions, chopped 1 teaspoon minced green garlic

Directions

Roast the chicken drumsticks in the preheated oven at 380 degrees F for 30 to 35 minutes. Add in the broccoli, celery, green onions, and green garlic. Add in the oregano, basil and olive oil; roast an additional 15 minutes. Bon appétit!

FISH AND SEAFOOD

105.   Easy Cod Fritters

(Ready in about 20 minutes | Servings 5) Per serving: 326 Calories; 21.7g Fat; 5.8g Carbs; 25.6g Protein; 1g Fiber

Ingredients

2 ½ cups cod fish, cooked 1/2 cup almond flour 1/2 cup Romano cheese, preferably freshly grated 3 tablespoons olive oil Sea salt and pepper, to taste 1 teaspoon butter, room temperature 1/2 teaspoon dried oregano 1/2 teaspoon dried thyme 1/4 cup onion, chopped 3 cups broccoli, cut into rice-sized chunks 2 eggs, whisked

Directions

Melt the butter in a pan over medium-high flame. Once hot, cook the broccoli for 5 to 6 minutes, until crisp-tender. Let it cool completely. Add in the cooked fish, salt, pepper, oregano, thyme, onion, eggs, almond flour, and cheese; mix until everything is well incorporated. Form the mixture into 10 patties. In a frying pan, heat the oil over a moderately high heat. Cook your fritters for 4 to 5 minutes per side.Bon appétit!

106.   Cod Fish Fillets with French Salad

(Ready in about 15 minutes + marinating time | Servings 4) Per serving: 425 Calories; 27.2g Fat; 6.1g Carbs; 38.3g Protein; 3g Fiber

Ingredients

4 white cod fish fillets 1 tablespoon olive oil 2 tablespoons fresh lemon juice 1 teaspoon garlic, minced 2 tablespoons scallions, chopped Salt and pepper, to taste For French Salad: 1 cup arugula 1 head Iceberg lettuce 2 tablespoons dandelion 1/4 cup red wine vinegar 1/4 cup extra-virgin olive oil 1 cup chicory 1 cup frissee Salt and ground black pepper, to your liking

Directions

Toss the cod fish fillets with the olive oil, lemon juice, garlic, scallions salt, and pepper; allow it to marinate for 2 hours in your refrigerator. Sear the fish fillets in the preheated skillet over moderately high heat; basting with the marinade. Toss all ingredients for the salad in a salad bowl.

107. Cheesy Salmon Dip

(Ready in about 10 minutes | Servings 10) Per serving: 109 Calories; 6.3g Fat; 1.3g Carbs; 11.4g Protein; 0.1g Fiber

Ingredients

10 ounces salmon 4 hard-boiled egg yolks, finely chopped 1/4 cup fresh scallions, chopped 5 ounces Ricotta cheese 5 ounces full-fat cream cheese Salt and freshly ground black pepper, to your liking 1/2 teaspoon hot paprika

Directions

Grill the salmon for about 10 minutes until browned and flakes easily with a fork. Cut into small chunks. Mix all ingredients until everything is well incorporated. Storing Place the cheesy salmon dip in airtight containers or Ziploc bags; keep in your refrigerator for up to 4 days.

108. Mediterranean-Style Tuna Salad with Bocconcini

(Ready in about 10 minutes | Servings 4) Per serving: 273 Calories; 11.7g Fat; 6.7g Carbs; 34.2g Protein; 4.1g Fiber

Ingredients

1 pound tuna steak 8 ounces bocconcini 1 teaspoon sesame oil 1 teaspoon balsamic vinegar 1 tablespoon fish sauce 1/2 cup radicchio, sliced 1 tomato, diced 1/2 cup black olives, pitted and sliced 2 teaspoons tahini paste 1/2 teaspoon chili pepper, finely chopped 1 head Romaine lettuce 2 garlic cloves, minced 1/2 cup onion, thinly sliced 2 bell peppers, sliced 1 Lebanese cucumber, sliced

Directions Grill the tuna over medium-high heat for about 4 minutes per side. Flake the fish with a fork. Mix the vegetables in a salad bowl. In a small mixing dish, thoroughly combine the tahini, sesame oil, vinegar, and fish sauce. Dress the salad.Enjoy!

109. Zingy Tuna Steaks with Spinach

(Ready in about 20 minutes | Servings 6) Per serving: 444 Calories; 38.2g Fat; 4.7g Carbs; 21.9g Protein; 1g Fiber

Ingredients

2 pounds tuna steaks 3 cups spinach 1 tablespoon Dijon mustard 3 tablespoons peanut oil Salt and pepper, to season 1/2 cup radishes, thinly sliced 1 fresh lemon, sliced 1 cup green onions, thinly sliced

Directions

Brush each tuna steaks with peanut oil and season them with salt and pepper. Arrange the tuna steaks on a foil-lined baking pan. Top with lemon slices, cover with foil and roast at 400 degrees F for about 10 minutes. Bon appétit!

110.   Mackerel and Vegetable Casserole

(Ready in about 30 minutes | Servings 4) Per serving: 301 Calories; 14g Fat; 6g Carbs; 33.3g Protein; 3.2g Fiber

Ingredients

1 pound mackerel steaks, chopped 1/2 stick butter Salt and black pepper, to your liking 1/4 cup fish consommé 1 cup goat cheese, shredded 1/2 cup fresh scallions, chopped 1/2 cup celery, thinly sliced 1 cup parsnip, thinly sliced 2 cloves garlic, thinly sliced 2 shallots, thinly sliced 2 tomatoes, thinly sliced

Directions

In a frying pan, melt the butter in over a moderately high heat. Cook the vegetables until they are just tender and fragrant. Add in the clam juice and tomatoes and cook for a further 5 minutes. Place the sautéed vegetables in a lightly-greased casserole dish. Lower the mackerel steaks on top of the vegetable layer. Sprinkle with salt and pepper. Bake in the preheated oven at 420 degrees F for about 15 minutes. Top with shredded cheese and bake for a further 5 to 6 minutes or until it is hot and bubbly. Bon appétit!

111. Clams with Garlic-Tomato Sauce

(Ready in about 25 minutes | Servings 4) Per serving: 134 Calories; 7.8g Fat; 5.9g Carbs; 8.3g Protein; 1g Fiber

Ingredients

40 littleneck clams For the Sauce: 2 tomatoes, pureed 2 tablespoons olive oil 1 shallot, chopped Sea salt and freshly ground black pepper, to taste 1/2 teaspoon paprika 1/3 cup port wine 2 garlic cloves, pressed 1/2 lemon, cut into wedges

Directions

Grill the clams until they are open, for 5 to 6 minutes. In a frying pan, heat the olive oil over moderate heat. Cook the shallot and garlic until tender and fragrant. Stir in the pureed tomatoes, salt, black pepper and paprika and continue to cook an additional 10 to 12 minutes or until thoroughly cooked. Heat off and add in the port wine; stir to combine. Garnish with fresh lemon wedges. Bon appétit!

112. Salad with Crispy-Skinned Snapper

(Ready in about 15 minutes | Servings 4) Per serving: 507 Calories; 42.8g Fat; 6g Carbs; 24.4g Protein; 2.7g Fiber

Ingredients

4 snapper fillets with skin 6 ounces Feta cheese, crumbled Sea salt and ground black pepper, to taste 1 teaspoon ground mustard seeds 1/2 teaspoon celery seeds 2 cups arugula 2 tablespoons butter, melted 2 cups lettuce leaves, torn into pieces 1 carrot, thinly sliced 1 cup spring onions, thinly sliced 1/2 cup black olives, pitted and sliced 10 grape tomatoes, halved For the Vinaigrette: 1/3 cup extra-virgin olive oil 1 teaspoon Dijon mustard 1 lime, juiced and zested 1 teaspoon ginger- garlic paste 1 teaspoon dried basil 2 tablespoons fresh mint, finely chopped Sea salt and ground black pepper, to taste

Directions

In a grill pan, melt the butter over a moderately high flame. Cook the fish for 5 to 6 minutes; flip the fish fillets over and cook them for 5 minutes more. Toss all ingredients for the salad. Whisk all ingredients for the vinaigrette and dress the salad.Top with the fish fillets, serve, and enjoy!

113. Red Snapper Soup

(Ready in about 20 minutes | Servings 4) Per serving: 316 Calories; 14.3g Fat; 6.6g Carbs; 32.7g Protein; 1.7g Fiber

Ingredients

1 pound red snapper, chopped 1 cup tomato puree 3 cups chicken stock 1/4 cup Marsala wine 2 thyme sprigs, chopped 1/2 teaspoon dried rosemary 1/2 stick butter, melted 1 medium leek, finely chopped 2 garlic cloves, minced 1/4 cup fresh parsley, chopped Sea salt and ground black pepper, to taste

Directions

In a heavy-bottomed pot, melt the butter over a moderately high heat. Cook the leek and garlic for 3 to 4 minutes or until tender and fragrant. Add in the parsley, tomato puree, chicken stock, wine, red snapper, and rosemary; bring to a rolling boil. Turn the heat to simmer; continue to simmer until the thoroughly cooked for a further 15 to 20 minutes. Season with salt and pepper to taste. Enjoy!

114. Rich and Spicy Seafood Stew

(Ready in about 25 minutes | Servings 4) Per serving: 296 Calories; 8.6g Fat; 5.5g Carbs; 41.4g Protein; 4.3g Fiber

Ingredients

1/2 pound sole, cut into 2-inch pieces 1/3 pound halibut, cut into 2-inch pieces 1/2 cup Marsala wine 1/8 teaspoon hot sauce, or more to taste 1 tablespoon lard, room temperature 1 cup shallots, chopped 1 teaspoon garlic, smashed Sea salt and black pepper, to taste 4 cups chicken bone broth 1 cup tomato sauce 2 thyme sprigs, chopped

Directions

In a large-sized pot, melt the lard over medium-high heat. Cook the shallots and garlic until they've softened. Add in the salt, black pepper, chicken bone broth, tomato sauce, and thyme and; continue to cook an additional 15 minutes. Add in the fish, wine and hot sauce; bring to a boil. Reduce the heat to simmer. Let it simmer for 4 to 5 minutes longer, stirring periodically. Enjoy!

115. Greek Salad with Grilled Halloumi

(Ready in about 15 minutes | Servings 4) Per serving: 199 Calories; 10.6g Fat; 6.1g Carbs; 14.2g Protein; 1.1g Fiber

Ingredients 1 pound halibut steak 1 cup cherry tomatoes, halved 1 onion, thinly sliced 1 tablespoon lemon juice 1 Lebanese cucumbers, thinly sliced 1/2 cup radishes, thinly sliced 2 tablespoons sunflower seeds 1 ½ tablespoons extra-virgin olive oil 1/2 head butterhead lettuce 1 cup Halloumi cheese Sea salt and pepper, to taste

Directions Cook the halibut steak on preheated grill for 5 to 6 minutes per side. until the fish flakes easily with a fork. Grill the halloumi cheese and slice into small pieces. Toss the grilled halloumi cheese with the remaining ingredients and set aside.Serve with chilled salad and enjoy!

116. Sour Cream Salmon with Parmesan

Ready in about: 25 minutes | Serves: 4 Per serving: Kcal 288, Fat 23.4g, Net Carbs 1.2g, Protein 16.2g

Ingredients 1 cup sour cream 1 tbsp fresh dill, chopped ½ lemon, zested and juiced Pink Salt and black pepper to taste 4 salmon steaks ½ cup Parmesan cheese, grated Preheat oven to 400°F.

DirectionsIn a bowl, mix the sour cream, dill, lemon zest, juice, salt, and pepper. Season the fish with salt and black pepper, drizzle lemon juice on both sides of the fish, and arrange them on a lined baking sheet. Spread the sour cream mixture on each fish and sprinkle with Parmesan cheese. Bake the fish for 15 minutes and after broil the top for 2 minutes with a close watch for a nice brown color. Plate the fish and serve with buttery green beans.

117. Steamed Salmon with Creamy Cucumber Sauce

Ready in about: 30 minutes | Serves: 4 Per serving: Kcal 458, Fat 30.4g, Net Carbs 2.6g, Protein 39.1g

Ingredients

4 salmon fillets, skin on 10 oz broccoli florets 2 tbsp olive oil 1 cucumber, diced 1 cup crème fraiche ¼ tsp lemon juice Salt and black pepper to taste 2 tbsp fresh dill

Directions

Combine the cucumber, crème fraiche, fresh dill, and lemon juice in a bowl. Season with salt and stir thoroughly. Cover and place in the refrigerator to chill until ready to use. Fill a large pot halfway up with water and place in a steamer basket; bring to a boil. Add in the broccoli florets and season with salt. Steam the broccoli for 6 minutes, until they are tender-crisp but still vibrant green. Transfer to a bowl and drizzle with olive oil; tent with foil to keep warm. Put the salmon in the basket, skin side down and sprinkle with salt and pepper. Cook for 8-10 minutes until the fish flakes easily. Serve the salmon topped with cucumber sauce and broccoli on the side.

118. Creamy Hoki with Almond Bread Crust

Ready in about: 50 minutes | Serves: 4 Per serving: Kcal 386, Fat 27g, Net Carbs 3.5g, Protein 28.5g

Ingredients

1 cup flaked smoked hoki, boneless 1 cup cubed hoki fillets, cubed 4 eggs 3 tbsp almond flour 1 onion, sliced 2 cups sour cream 1 tbsp chopped parsley 1 cup pork rinds, crushed 1 cup grated cheddar cheese Salt and black pepper to taste 2 tbsp butter

Directions

Boil the eggs in salted water in a pot over medium heat for 10 minutes. Run the eggs under cold water and peel the shells. After, place on a cutting board and chop them. Melt the butter in a saucepan over medium heat and sauté the onion for 4 minutes. Turn the heat off and stir in the almond flour to form a roux. Turn the heat back on and cook the roux until golden brown and stir in the sour cream until the mixture is smooth. Season with salt and pepper and stir in the parsley. Preheat oven to 360°F. Spread the smoked and cubed fish on a greased baking dish, sprinkle the eggs on top, and spoon the sauce over. In a bowl, mix pork rinds and cheddar cheese and spread over the sauce. Bake the casserole in the oven for 20 minutes until the top is golden and the sauce and cheese are bubbly. Remove the bake after and serve with a steamed green vegetable mix.

119.Blackened Fish Tacos with Slaw

Ready in about: 20 minutes | Serves: 4 Per serving: Kcal 268, Fat: 20g, Net Carbs: 3.5g, Protein: 13.8g

Ingredients

1 tbsp olive oil 1 tsp chili powder 2 tilapia fillets 1 tsp paprika 4 low carb tortillas Slaw ½ cup red cabbage, shredded 1 tbsp lemon juice 1 tsp apple cider vinegar 1 tbsp olive oil Salt and black pepper to taste

Directions

Season the tilapia with chili powder and paprika. Heat the olive oil in a skillet over medium heat. Add tilapia and cook until blackened, about 3 minutes per side. Cut into strips. Divide the tilapia between the tortillas. Combine all slaw ingredients in a bowl and top the fish to serve.

120.   Sicilian-Style Sardines with Zoodles

Ready in about: 10 minutes | Serves: 2 Per serving: Kcal 355, Fat: 31g, Net Carbs: 6g, Protein: 20g

Ingredients

4 cups zoodles (zucchini spirals) 2 oz cubed bacon 4 oz canned sardines, chopped ½ cup canned tomatoes, chopped 1 tbsp capers 1 garlic clove, minced

Directions

Pour some of the sardine oil into a pan over medium heat. Add the garlic and sauté for 1 minute. Stir in bacon and cook for 2 more minutes. Pour in the tomatoes and simmer for 5 minutes. Add zoodles and sardines and cook for 3 minutes. Transfer to a serving plate and top with capers. Serve.

121.Cod in Garlic Butter Sauce

Ready in about: 20 minutes | Serves: 6 Per serving: Kcal 264, Fat 17.3g, Net Carbs 2.3g, Protein 20g

Ingredients

2 tsp olive oil 6 Alaska cod fillets Salt and black pepper to taste 4 tbsp butter 3 cloves garlic, minced ⅓ cup lemon juice 3 tbsp white wine 2 tbsp chopped chives Heat the oil in a skillet over medium heat.

DirectionsSeason the cod with salt and black pepper. Fry the fillets in the oil for 4 minutes on one side, flip, and cook for 1 minute. Take out, plate, and set aside. In the same skillet over, Melt the butter and sauté the garlic for 3 minutes. Add the lemon juice, white wine, and chives. Season with salt and black pepper and cook for 3 minutes until the wine slightly reduces. Put the fish in a platter, spoon the sauce over, and serve with buttered green beans.

122.   Coconut Crab Patties

Ready in about: 15 minutes | Serves: 4 Per serving: Kcal 215, Fat: 11.5g, Net Carbs: 3.6g, Protein: 15.3g

Ingredients

2 tbsp coconut oil 1 tbsp lemon juice 1 lb lump crab meat 2 tsp Dijon mustard 1 egg, beaten 1 ½ tbsp coconut flour

DirectionsIn a bowl, add all the ingredients except the oil and mix well. Make patties out of the mixture. Melt the coconut oil in a skillet over medium heat. Add the crab patties and cook for about 2-3 minutes per side.

123.   Lemon Garlic Shrimp

Ready in about: 22 minutes | Serves: 6 Per serving: Kcal 258, Fat 22g, Net Carbs 2g, Protein 13g

Ingredients

½ cup butter, divided 2 lb shrimp, peeled and deveined Salt and black pepper to taste ¼ tsp sweet paprika 3 garlic cloves, minced 1 lemon, zested and juiced

DirectionsMelt the butter in a skillet over medium heat. Season the shrimp with salt, pepper, and paprika and add to the butter. Cook for 4 minutes on both sides until pink. Set aside. Include the lemon zest, juice, garlic, and 3 tbsp water to the skillet. Return the shrimp and cook for 2 minutes. Serve warm.

124.   Italian-Style Seafood Stew

(Ready in about 20 minutes | Servings 4) Per serving: 209 Calories; 12.6g Fat; 6.6g Carbs; 15.2g Protein; 2g Fiber

Ingredients

2 tablespoons lard, room temperature 1/2 teaspoon lime zest 1/2 pound shrimp 1/2 pound scallops 1 teaspoon Italian seasonings blend Salt and ground black pepper, to taste 1 leek, chopped 2 garlic cloves, pressed 1 cup tomato puree 1 celery stalk, chopped 3 cups fish stock 2 tablespoons port wine

Directions

Melt the lard in a large pot over a moderately high heat. Sauté the leek and garlic until they've softened. Stir in the pureed tomatoes and continue to cook for about 10 minutes. Add in the remaining ingredients and bring to a boil. Turn the heat to a simmer and continue to cook for 4 to 5 minutes. Enjoy!

125. Creole Tuna with Lemon

(Ready in about 40 minutes | Servings 4) Per serving: 266 Calories; 11.5g Fat; 5.6g Carbs; 34.9g Protein; 0.7g Fiber

Ingredients

4 tuna fillets 1/4 cup scallions, chopped 2 garlic cloves, minced 1/3 cup fresh lemon juice 1/3 cup coconut aminos 3 teaspoons olive oil 1 teaspoon lemon thyme Salt and ground black pepper 1 teaspoon dried rosemary

Directions

Place all ingredients in a ceramic dish; cover and let it marinate for about 30 minutes in the refrigerator. Grill the tuna fillets for about 15 minutes, basting with the reserved marinade.

126. Pepper Boats with Herring

(Ready in about 10 minutes | Servings 4) Per serving: 120 Calories; 5.4g Fat; 5.8g Carbs; 12.3g Protein; 1.6g Fiber

Ingredients

4 pickled peppers, slice into halves 8 ounces canned herring, drained 1 teaspoon Dijon mustard 1 celery, chopped 1 cup onions, chopped Salt and freshly ground black pepper, to taste 1 tablespoon fresh coriander, chopped

Directions

Broil the bell pepper for 5 to 6 minutes until they've softened. Cut into halves and discard the seeds. In a mixing bowl, thoroughly combine the herring, Dijon mustard, celery, onions, salt, black pepper, and fresh coriander. Mix to combine well. Spoon the mixture into the bell pepper halves.Reheat the thawed peppers at 200 degrees F until they are completely warm. Enjoy!

127.Old-Fashioned Seafood Chowder

(Ready in about 15 minutes | Servings 5) Per serving: 404 Calories; 30g Fat; 5.3g Carbs; 23.9g Protein; 0.3g Fiber

Ingredients 1/2 stick butter 3/4 pound prawns, peeled and deveined 1/2 pound crab meat 2 tablespoons scallions, chopped 1 tablespoon tomato sauce 1 teaspoon Mediterranean spice mix 1 egg, lightly beaten 2 garlic cloves, minced 1/3 cup port wine 1 quart chicken bone broth 2 cups double cream

Directions In a heavy bottomed pot, melt the butter over a moderately high flame. Sauté the scallions and garlic until they've softened. Add in the prawns, crab meat, wine, and chicken bone broth. Continue to cook until thoroughly heated for 5 to 6 minutes. Decrease the heat to low; add in the remaining ingredients and continue to simmer for 5 minutes more.Enjoy!

128.   Chinese-Style Mackerel Chowder

(Ready in about 30 minutes | Servings 6) Per serving: 165 Calories; 5.5g Fat; 4g Carbs; 25.4g Protein; 0.5g Fiber

Ingredients 1 ¼ pounds mackerel, cut into small pieces 1 tablespoon peanut oil 1 chili pepper, deveined and sliced 1 tablespoon coconut aminos 1/4 cup fresh mint, chopped 2 ½ cups hot water 1 teaspoon Five-spice powder 1/2 cup white onions, sliced 1 garlic clove, smashed 1 celery rib, diced 1 bell pepper, deveined and sliced 3/4 cup heavy cream

Directions

Heat the oil in a large pot over a moderately high heat. Cook the onion and garlic until they are just tender or about 3 minutes. Stir in the celery, peppers, coconut aminos, water, and Five-spice powder. Reduce to a simmer, and cook, partially covered, for 15 minutes. Fold in the fish chunks and continue to simmer an additional 15 minutes or until cooked through. Add in the heavy cream and remove from heat.Serve with fresh mint leaves and enjoy!

129.   Colorful Prawn Salad

(Ready in about 10 minutes + chilling time | Servings 6) Per serving: 209 Calories; 9.5g Fat; 6.8g Carbs; 20.2g Protein; 0.4g Fiber

Ingredients 1 medium-sized lemon, cut into wedges 2 pounds prawns 1/2 cup mayonnaise 1/2 cup cream cheese 1/2 teaspoon stone-ground mustard 1 tablespoon dry sherry 1 tablespoon balsamic vinegar Salt and black pepper 4 scallion stalks, chopped 1 Italian pepper, sliced 1 cucumber, sliced 1 ½ cups radishes, sliced 1 tablespoon Sriracha sauce

Directions Bring a pot of a lightly salted water to a boil over high heat. Add in the lemon and prawns and cook approximately 3 minutes, until they are opaque. Drain and rinse your prawns. In a salad bowl, toss the remaining ingredients until well combined.Top with the prepared prawns and serve!

130.   Salmon and Ricotta Stuffed Tomatoes

(Ready in about 30 minutes | Servings 6) Per serving: 303 Calories; 22.9g Fat; 6.8g Carbs; 17g Protein; 1.6g Fiber

Ingredients 6 tomatoes, pulp and seeds removed 1 ½ cups Ricotta cheese 10 ounces salmon 1 cup scallions, finely chopped 2 garlic cloves, minced 2 tablespoons coriander, chopped 1/2 cup aioli 1 teaspoon Dijon mustard Sea salt and ground black pepper, to taste

Directions Grill your salmon for about 10 minutes until browned and flakes easily with a fork. Cut into small chunks. Thoroughly combine the salmon, scallions, garlic, coriander, aioli, mustard, salt, and pepper in a bowl. Spoon the filling into tomatoes. Bake in the preheated oven at 390 degrees F for 17 to 20 minutes until they are thoroughly cooked.Enjoy!

131. Haddock and Vegetable Skewers

(Ready in about 15 minutes | Servings 4) Per serving: 257 Calories; 12.5g Fat; 7g Carbs; 27.5g Protein; 0.9g Fiber

Ingredients

1 pound haddock, cut into small cubes Salt and pepper, to taste 1/2 teaspoon basil 2 tablespoons olive oil 1 red onion, cut into wedges 1 zucchini, diced 1 cup cherry tomatoes 2 tablespoons coconut aminos

Directions

Start by preheating your grill on high. Toss the haddock and vegetables with salt, pepper, basil, olive oil, and coconut aminos. Alternate the seasoned haddock, onion, zucchini and tomatoes on bamboo skewers. Grill your skewers for 5 minutes for medium-rare, flipping them occasionally to ensure even cooking. Bon appétit!

132. Avocado and Shrimp Salad

(Ready in about 10 minutes + chilling time | Servings 6) Per serving: 236 Calories; 14.3g Fat; 5.3g Carbs; 16.3g Protein; 3g Fiber

Ingredients

1 cup butterhead lettuce 1 avocado, pitted and sliced 1/2 cup aioli 1 pound shrimp, peeled and deveined 1/2 cup cucumber, chopped 1 shallot, thinly sliced 1 tablespoon soy sauce 2 teaspoons fresh lemon juice

Directions

Cook your shrimp in a pot of salted water for about 3 minutes. Drain and reserve. In a salad bowl, mix all ingredients, except for the lettuce leaves. Gently stir to combine. Enjoy!

133. Classic Fish Tart

(Ready in about 45 minutes | Servings 6) Per serving: 416 Calories; 34.2g Fat; 5.5g Carbs; 19.5g Protein; 1.5g Fiber

Ingredients

For the Crust: 1 teaspoon baking powder Flaky salt, to taste 1/2 stick butter 1 cup almond meal 3 tablespoons flaxseed meal 2 teaspoons ground psyllium husk powder 2 eggs 2 tablespoons almond milk For the Filling: 10 ounces cod fish, chopped 2 eggs 1 teaspoon Mediterranean spice mix 1 ½ cups Colby cheese, shredded 1 teaspoon stone-ground mustard 1/2 cup cream cheese 1/2 cup mayonnaise

Directions Thoroughly combine all the crust ingredients. Press the crust into a parchment-lined baking pan. Bake the crust in the preheated oven at 365 degrees F for about 15 minutes. In a mixing dish, combine the ingredients for the filling. Spread the mixture over the pie crust and bake for a further 25 minutes. Enjoy!

134.　Trout with Authentic Chimichurri Sauce

(Ready in about 15 minutes | Servings 6) Per serving: 265 Calories; 20.9g Fat; 4g Carbs; 17.1g Protein; 0.7g Fiber

Ingredients

2 tablespoons butter 6 trout fillets Sea salt and ground black pepper, to taste 1/2 teaspoon curry powder 1/2 teaspoon mustard seeds For Chimichurri Sauce: 1/3 cup apple cider vinegar Kosher salt and pepper, to taste 2 garlic cloves, minced 1/2 cup yellow onion, finely chopped 1 chili pepper, finely chopped 1/2 cup fresh cilantro, minced 1 tablespoon fresh basil leaves, snipped 1/3 cup olive oil

Directions

In a cast-iron skillet, melt the butter over a moderately high heat. Season the trout fillets with salt, pepper, curry powder, and mustard seeds. Cook the trout fillets for about 5 minutes per side. To make the Chimichurri sauce, pulse the remaining ingredients in your food processor until well mixed.

135.　Herby Salmon in Creamy Sauce

Ready in about: 15 minutes | Serves: 2 Per serving: Kcal 468, Fat: 40g, Net Carbs: 1.5g, Protein: 22g

Ingredients

2 salmon fillets 1 tsp dried tarragon 1 tsp dried dill 3 tbsp butter ¼ cup heavy cream Salt and black pepper to taste

Directions

Season the salmon with some dill and tarragon. Warm butter in a pan over medium heat. Add salmon and cook for 4 minutes on both sides. Set aside. In the same pan, add the remaining dill and tarragon. Cook for 30 seconds to infuse the flavors. Whisk in the heavy cream, season with salt and black pepper, and cook for 2-3 minutes. Serve the salmon topped with the sauce.

136.   Trout & Fennel Parcels

Ready in about: 20 minutes | Serves: 4 Per serving: Kcal 234, Fat 9.3g, Net Carbs 2.8g, Protein 17g

Ingredients

1 lb deboned trout, butterflied Salt and black pepper to taste 3 tbsp olive oil + extra for tossing 4 sprigs thyme 4 butter cubes 1 fennel bulb, thinly sliced 1 medium red onion, sliced 8 lemon slices 3 tsp capers Preheat oven to 400°F.

Directions

Cut out parchment paper wide enough for each trout. In a bowl, toss the fennel and onion with a little bit of olive oil and share into the middle parts of the papers. Place the fish on each veggie mound, top with a drizzle of olive oil each, salt, pepper, 1 sprig of thyme, and 1 cube of butter. Lay the lemon slices on the fish. Wrap and close the packets securely and place them on a baking sheet. Bake in the oven for 15 minutes. Garnish the fish with capers and serve.

137.Tuna Steaks with Shirataki Noodles

Ready in about: 30 minutes | Serves: 4 Per serving: Kcal 310, Fat 18.2g, Net Carbs 2g, Protein 22g

Ingredients

1 pack (7 oz) miracle noodle angel hair 1 red bell pepper, seeded and halved 4 tuna steaks Salt and black pepper to taste 2 tbsp olive oil 2 tbsp pickled ginger 2 tbsp chopped cilantro 1 tbsp olive oil

Dircctions

In a colander, rinse the shirataki noodles with running cold water. Bring a pot of salted water to a boil. Blanch the noodles for 2 minutes. Drain and transfer to a dry skillet over medium heat. Dry roast for a minute until opaque. Grease a grill grate with olive oil and preheat to medium heat. Season the red bell pepper and tuna with salt and pepper, brush with olive oil, and grill covered for 3 minutes on each side. Transfer to a plate to cool. Assemble the noodles, tuna, and bell pepper into a serving platter. Top with pickled ginger and garnish with cilantro. Serve with roasted sesame sauce.

138.   Salmon Panzanella

Ready in about: 22 minutes | Serves: 4 Per serving: Kcal 338, Fat 21.7g, Net Carbs 3.1g, Protein 28.5g

Ingredients

1 lb skinned salmon, cut into 4 steaks each 1 cucumber, peeled, seeded, cubed Salt and black pepper to taste 8 black olives, pitted and chopped 1 tbsp capers, rinsed 2 large tomatoes, diced 3 tbsp red wine vinegar ¼ cup red onion, thinly sliced 3 tbsp olive oil 2 slices zero carb bread, cubed Preheat a grill to 350°F.

Directions

In a bowl, mix the cucumber, olives, pepper, capers, tomatoes, wine vinegar, onion, olive oil, and bread. Let sit for a few minutes to incorporate the flavors. Season the salmon with salt and pepper. Grill them on both sides for 8 minutes in total. Serve the salmon with the veggies' salad.

139.   Tilapia with Olives & Tomato Sauce

Ready in about: 30 minutes | Serves: 4 Per serving: Kcal 282, Fat: 15g, Net Carbs: 6g, Protein: 23g

Ingredients

4 tilapia fillets 2 garlic cloves, minced ½ tsp dried oregano 14 oz canned tomatoes, diced 2 tbsp olive oil ½ red onion, chopped 2 tbsp fresh parsley, chopped ¼ cup Kalamata olives

Directions

Heat olive oil in a skillet over medium heat and cook the onion for 3 minutes. Add garlic and oregano and cook for 30 seconds. Stir in tomatoes and bring the mixture to a boil. Reduce the heat and simmer for 5 minutes. Add olives and tilapia and cook for about 8 minutes. Serve the tilapia with tomato sauce.

140.   Grilled Shrimp with Chimichurri Sauce

Ready in about: 10 minutes + marinating time | Serves: 4 Per serving: Kcal 283, Fat: 20.3g, Net Carbs: 3.5g, Protein: 16g

Ingredients

1 lb shrimp, peeled and deveined 2 tbsp olive oil Juice of 1 lime Chimichurri ½ tsp salt ¼ cup olive oil 2 garlic cloves ¼ cup red onions, chopped ¼ cup red wine vinegar ½ tsp pepper 2 cups parsley ¼ tsp red pepper flakes

Directions Process the chimichurri ingredients in a blender until smooth; set aside. Combine the shrimp, olive oil, and lime juice in a bowl. Let marinate in the fridge for 30 minutes. Preheat the grill to medium heat. Add shrimp and cook for about 2 minutes per side. Serve shrimp drizzled with the chimichurri sauce.

141. Shrimp in Curry Sauce

Ready in about: 15 minutes | Serves: 2 Per serving: Kcal 560, Fat: 41g, Net Carbs: 4.3g, Protein: 24.4g

Ingredients

½ oz Parmesan cheese, grated 1 egg, beaten ¼ tsp curry powder 2 tsp almond flour ½ lb shrimp, shelled 3 tbsp coconut oil Sauce 2 tbsp curry leaves 2 tbsp butter ½ onion, diced ½ cup heavy cream ½ oz cheddar cheese, shredded

Directions

Combine all dry ingredients for the batter. Melt the coconut oil in a skillet over medium heat. Dip the shrimp in the egg first, and then coat with the dry mixture. Fry until golden and crispy, about 5-6 minutes. Melt the butter in the skillet. Add onion and cook for 3 minutes. Stir in curry leaves for 30 seconds. Mix in heavy cream and cheddar cheese and cook until thickened, 2 minutes. Add shrimp. Stir to coat. Serve.

142. Coconut Curry Mussels

Ready in about: 25 minutes | Serves: 6 Per serving: Kcal 356, Fat 20.6g, Net Carbs 0.3g, Protein 21.1g

Ingredients

3 lb mussels, cleaned, de-bearded 1 cup minced shallots 3 tbsp minced garlic 1 ½ cups coconut milk 2 cups dry white wine 2 tsp red curry powder ⅓ cup coconut oil ⅓ cup chopped green onions ⅓ cup chopped parsley

Directions

Pour the wine into a saucepan and cook the shallots and garlic over medium heat, 5 minutes. Stir in the coconut milk and red curry powder and cook for 3 minutes. Add the mussels and steam for 7 minutes or until their shells are opened. Then, use a slotted spoon to remove to a bowl leaving the sauce in the pan. Discard any closed mussels at this point. Stir the coconut oil into the sauce, turn the heat off, and stir in the parsley and green onions. Serve the mussels immediately with a butternut squash mash.

143.   Cheesy Tuna Pâté

(Ready in about 10 minutes | Servings 6) Per serving: 181 Calories; 10.4g Fat; 2.1g Carbs; 19g Protein; 1g Fiber

Ingredients

2 (6-ounce) cans tuna in oil, drained 1 tablespoon fresh Italian parsley, chopped 1/2 cup Cottage cheese 1 ounce sunflower seeds, ground 1 ounce sesame seeds, ground 1/2 teaspoon mustard seeds

Directions

Add all of the above ingredients to a bowl of your blender or food processor. Blend until everything is well combined.

144.   Old Bay Sea Bass Chowder

(Ready in about 30 minutes | Servings 4) Per serving: 170 Calories; 5.8g Fat; 5.7g Carbs; 20g Protein; 1.9g Fiber

Ingredients

1 ¼ pounds sea bass, skin removed, cut into small chunks 2 carrots, chopped 1/4 cup port wine 1/2 cup sour cream Sea salt and ground black pepper, to taste 1 teaspoon Old Bay seasonings 3 teaspoons olive oil 1 onion, chopped 1 celery rib, chopped 3 cups boiling water 1/2 cup fish stock

Directions In a heavy-bottomed pot, heat the olive oil over a moderately high flame. Once hot, cook the fish for about 10. Stir in the onion, celery, carrot, spices, water, and fish stock and bring to a boil. Turn the heat to medium-low. Let it simmer for 15 to 20 minutes more or until thoroughly cooked. Afterwards, add in the port wine and sour cream. Remove form the heat and stir to combine well.Bon appétit!

145.   Swordfish with Mashed Cauliflower

(Ready in about 35 minutes | Servings 4) Per serving: 404 Calories; 22.2g Fat; 5.7g Carbs; 43.5g Protein; 3g Fiber

Ingredients 1 ½ tablespoons extra-virgin olive oil 1 tablespoon freshly squeezed lemon juice 1 pound swordfish cutlets, about 3/4 inch thick 1/2 cup fresh basil, roughly chopped Flaky sea salt and ground black pepper, to taste 1 ½ teaspoons Greek herb mix 1/4 cup Romano cheese, freshly grated 1 pound cauliflower, broken into florets 1/4 cup double cream 2 tablespoons butter

Directions Whisk the extra-virgin olive oil with the lemon juice. Grill the fish cutlets for about 15 minutes, basting them with the lemon mixture. Season with salt, black pepper, and Greek herb mix. Reserve, keeping them warm. Boil the cauliflower in a lightly salted water until crisp-tender. Mash the cauliflower with a potato masher. Fold in the other ingredients and stir to combine well.

146.   Easy Halibut Steaks

(Ready in about 35 minutes | Servings 2) Per serving: 308 Calories; 10.9g Fat; 2g Carbs; 46.5g Protein; 0.8g Fiber

Ingredients

2 halibut steaks 1 teaspoon garlic, finely minced 1/3 cup freshly squeezed lime juice 1 teaspoon dry rosemary 1 teaspoon dry thyme 4 tablespoons fresh chives, chopped 2 teaspoons sesame oil, room temperature Flaky sea salt and white pepper, to taste

Directions

Place the fresh lime juice, sesame oil, salt, white pepper, rosemary, thyme, chives, garlic, and halibut steak in a ceramic dish; let it marinate for about 30 minutes. Grill the halibut steaks approximately 15 minutes, turning occasionally and basting with the reserved marinade.Bon appétit!

147.   Sherry and Butter Prawns

(Ready in about 10 minutes + marinating time | Servings 4) Per serving: 294 Calories; 14.3g Fat; 3.6g Carbs; 34.6g Protein; 1.4g Fiber

Ingredients 1 ½ pounds king prawns, peeled and deveined 2 tablespoons dry sherry 1 teaspoon dried basil 1/2 teaspoon mustard seeds 1 ½ tablespoons fresh lemon juice 1 teaspoon cayenne pepper, crushed 1 tablespoon garlic paste 1/2 stick butter, at room temperature

Directions Whisk the dry sherry with cayenne pepper, garlic paste, basil, mustard seeds, lemon juice and prawns. Let it marinate for 1 hour in your refrigerator. In a frying pan, melt the butter over medium-high flame, basting with the reserved marinade. Sprinkle with salt and pepper to taste. Enjoy!

148.   Super Easy Fish Cakes

(Ready in about 30 minutes | Servings 6) Per serving: 234 Calories; 10.6g Fat; 2.5g Carbs; 31.2g Protein; 0.2g Fiber

Ingredients

1 ½ pounds tilapia fish, deboned and flaked 2 tablespoons sesame oil 1/2 cup Cottage cheese, at room temperature 2 eggs, lightly beaten 1/4 cup almond meal 1/4 tablespoons flax meal 2 teaspoons brown mustard Sea salt and pepper, to taste 2 tablespoons fresh basil, chopped

Directions

Mix the flakes fish with the eggs, almond and flax meal, cheese, mustard, salt, pepper, and basil. Form the mixture into 12 patties. Now, place the patties on a parchment-lined baking sheet. Spritz them with sesame oil. Bake in the preheated oven at 395 degrees F approximately 25 minutes, rotating the pan occasionally once. Bon appétit!

149. Crabmeat and Vegetable Bowl

(Ready in about 10 minutes | Servings 4) Per serving: 232 Calories; 15.6g Fat; 6g Carbs; 18.9g Protein; 2g Fiber

Ingredients

12 ounces lump legs 10 Kalamata olives, pitted and halved 1/4 cup fresh scallions, chopped 2 ounces thinly sliced bacon, chopped 4 cups spinach 1 large-sized tomato, diced 3 tablespoons olive oil 1 tablespoon peanut butter 1/2 lime, zested and juiced Flaky sea salt and ground black pepper, to your liking 1/4 cup fresh parsley, chopped

Directions

Start by preheating your grill to 225 degrees F for indirect cooking. Place the crab legs on the grill grates. Close the lid and grill for about 30 minutes or until done. To prepare the dressing, whisk the oil, peanut butter, lime juice, salt, and pepper. Toss the remaining ingredients and dress your salad. Bon appétit!

150. Creamed Halibut Fillets with Brown Mushrooms

(Ready in about 20 minutes | Servings 4) Per serving: 585 Calories; 30.5g Fat; 5.5g Carbs; 66.8g Protein; 1.1g Fiber

Ingredients

4 halibut fillets 1 ½ cups chicken stock 1/2 cup fresh scallions, chopped 1 cup sour cream 2 tablespoons olive oil 1 medium-sized leek, chopped 1/2 pound brown mushrooms, thinly sliced 2 garlic cloves, chopped Sea salt and freshly ground black pepper, to taste 1 tablespoon butter

Directions

Heat the olive oil in a saucepan over a moderately high heat. Cook the leek until tender and translucent. Add in the mushrooms, garlic, salt, and black pepper and continue to cook for 5 minutes more or until the mushrooms release liquid. Add in the halibut fillets and continue to cook over medium-high heat approximately 5 minutes on each side. Add in the butter, chicken stock, and scallions; bring to a boil. Immediately reduce the heat and let it cook for 10 minutes more or until heated through. Add in the sour cream, remove from the heat and stir to combine well.Bon appétit!

151. Amberjack Fillets with Cheese Sauce

(Ready in about 20 minutes | Servings 6) Per serving: 285 Calories; 20.4g Fat; 1.2g Carbs; 23.8g Protein; 0.1g Fiber

Ingredients

6 amberjack fillets 1/4 cup fresh tarragon chopped 2 tablespoons olive oil, at room temperature Sea salt and ground black pepper, to taste For the Sauce: 1/3 cup vegetable broth 3/4 cup double cream 1/3 cup Romano cheese, grated 3 teaspoons butter, at room temperature 2 garlic cloves, finely minced

Directions

In a non-stick frying pan, heat the olive oil until sizzling. Once hot, fry the amberjack for about 6 minutes per side or until the edges are turning opaque. Sprinkle them with salt, black pepper, and tarragon. Reserve. To make the sauce, melt the butter in a saucepan over moderately high heat. Sauté the garlic until tender and fragrant or about 2 minutes. Add in the vegetable broth and cream and continue to cook for 5 to 6 minutes more; heat off. Stir in the Romano cheese and continue stirring in the residual heat for a couple of minutes more.Bon appétit!

152. Refreshing Prawn Salad

(Ready in about 10 minutes | Servings 6) Per serving: 196 Calories; 8.3g Fat; 6.5g Carbs; 21.4g Protein; 1.6g Fiber

Ingredients

2 pounds tiger prawns, peeled leaving tails intact Sea salt and freshly ground black pepper, to taste 1 celery rib, sliced 1 cup white onions, chopped 1 Lebanese cucumber, chopped 1/2 head Iceberg lettuce, torn into pieces 1/4 cup fresh basil, chopped Juice from 1 fresh lime 1/4 cup capers, drained 1/2 cup mayonnaise

Directions

Boil the tiger prawns in a large pot of salted water for about 3 minutes. Drain well and let it cool completely. Toss the remaining ingredients in a large bowl; toss to combine well. Top with the tiger prawns and serve immediately!

153. Family Seafood Bowl

(Ready in about 10 minutes | Servings 4) Per serving: 260 Calories; 13.6g Fat; 5.9g Carbs; 28.1g Protein; 1.5g Fiber

Ingredients

1 pound sea scallops, halved horizontally 1/2 cup Kalamata olives, pitted and sliced 2 cups arugula 1/2 tablespoon Dijon mustard 1 teaspoon garlic, chopped 1 cup cherry tomatoes, halved 1 Lebanese cucumber, sliced 1/4 cup extra-virgin olive oil 2 tablespoons fresh lime juice Sea salt and pepper, to season

Directions Boil the scallops in a pot of a lightly salted water for about 3 minutes or until opaque; place them in a serving bowl. To make the salad, toss the remaining ingredients until everything is well combined.. Enjoy!

154. Avocado and Herring Fat Bombs

(Ready in about 5 minutes | Servings 4) Per serving: 316 Calories; 24.4g Fat; 5.9g Carbs; 17.4g Protein; 4.2g Fiber

Ingredients

1 avocado, pitted and peeled 1/2 cup scallions, chopped 1 teaspoon capers 1 can herring Salt and black pepper, to taste 3 ounces sunflower seeds 1/2 teaspoon hot paprika

Directions In a mixing bowl, combine all ingredients until well incorporated. Roll the mixture into 8 balls.Bon appétit!

155. Smoky Sardine Salad

(Ready in about 10 minutes | Servings 4) Per serving: 195 Calories; 14.7g Fat; 6g Carbs; 7.8g Protein; 3.1g Fiber

Ingredients

1 head of Iceberg lettuce 1 pound fresh sardines, chopped 1 red onion, chopped 1 celery, thinly sliced 1/2 cup cucumber, thinly sliced Sea salt and ground black pepper, to taste 3/4 cup mayonnaise 1/2 teaspoon smoked paprika 1/4 cup fresh scallions, roughly chopped

Directions Pat your sardines dry with a kitchen paper towel. Place your sardines in a baking dish; roast them in the preheated oven at 390 degrees F for 20 minutes. Toss the remaining ingredients in a salad bowl.Top your salad with the sardines and enjoy!

VEGETARIAN,SOUP STEW AND SALAD

156. Summer Cheese Ball

(Ready in about 25 minutes | Servings 2) Per serving: 133 Calories; 9.9g Fat; 6.8g Carbs; 6g Protein; 0.7g Fiber

Ingredients

1 Lebanese cucumber, chopped 2 tablespoons pine nuts, chopped 1 teaspoon salt 1 ounce Feta cheese 1 ounce Neufchatel 1 tablespoon fresh basil, chopped

Directions

Salt the chopped cucumber and place it in a colander. Let it stand for 30 minutes; press the cucumber to drain away the excess liquid and transfer to a mixing bowl. Mix in the cheese and basil. Shape the mixture into a ball and top with chopped nuts.Enjoy!

157.Greek-Style Roasted Asparagus

(Ready in about 15 minutes | Servings 6) Per serving: 128 Calories; 9.4g Fat; 2.9g Carbs; 6.4g Protein; 2.9g Fiber

Ingredients 1 cup Halloumi cheese, crumbled 1 red onion, chopped 2 garlic cloves, minced 1 ½ pounds asparagus spears 2 tablespoons extra-virgin olive oil Salt and black pepper, to the taste

Directions

Brush your asparagus with extra-virgin olive oil. Toss with the onion, garlic, salt, and black pepper. Roast in the preheated oven at 395 degrees F for about 15 minutes.Enjoy!

158. Cheddar and Mushroom-Stuffed Peppers

(Ready in about 30 minutes | Servings 6) Per serving: 319 Calories; 18.8g Fat; 5.6g Carbs; 10.3g Protein; 1.9g Fiber

Ingredients 6 bell peppers, seeds and tops removed 1/2 cup Cheddar cheese, grated ½ cup tomato puree 3/4 pound Cremini mushrooms, chopped 2 tablespoons olive oil 1 onion, chopped 1 teaspoon garlic, minced 2 tablespoons fresh cilantro, chopped 1 teaspoon mustard seeds Salt to taste

Directions In a frying pan, heat the olive oil over a moderately-high flame. Sauté the onion and garlic until they are tender and aromatic. Add in the Cremini mushrooms and continue to cook for a further 5 minutes or until the mushrooms release the liquid. Add in the cilantro, mustard seeds, and salt; stir to combine. Divide this filling between bell peppers. Place the peppers in a lightly greased casserole dish. Pour the tomato sauce around stuffed peppers. Bake at 385 degrees F for about 22 minutes or until heated through.

159.   Creole Cheesy Spinach

(Ready in about 10 minutes | Servings 4) Per serving: 208 Calories; 13.5g Fat; 6g Carbs; 14.5g Protein; 5.1g Fiber

Ingredients

2 pounds spinach, torn into pieces 1/2 stick butter Sea salt and pepper, to taste 1/4 teaspoon caraway seeds 1 cup Creole cream cheese 1 teaspoon garlic, pressed

Directions

Melt the butter in a saucepan over medium-high heat; now, sauté the garlic until tender and fragrant. Add the spinach, salt, pepper, and caraway seeds; continue to cook for about 6 minutes until warmed through.Enjoy!

160.   Spicy and Aromatic Chinese Cabbage

(Ready in about 15 minutes | Servings 4) Per serving: 53 Calories; 3.7g Fat; 3.2g Carbs; 1.7g Protein; 2.1g Fiber

Ingredients

3/4 pound Chinese cabbage, cored and cut into chunks 1 teaspoon Chinese Five-spice powder Salt and Sichuan pepper, to taste 1 tablespoon sesame oil 1 shallot, sliced 1/2 teaspoon chili sauce, sugar-free 2 tablespoons rice wine 1 tablespoon soy sauce

Directions

Heat the sesame oil in a wok a moderately-high heat. Sauté the shallot until tender and translucent. Add in the Chinese cabbage and continue to cook for about 3 minutes. Partially cover and add in the remaining ingredients; continue to cook for 5 minutes more.Bon appétit!

161.Old-Fashioned Cabbage with Bacon and Eggs

(Ready in about 15 minutes | Servings 4) Per serving: 173 Calories; 10.6g Fat; 5.6g Carbs; 14.2g Protein; 1.6g Fiber

Ingredients

2 cups cabbage, shredded 2 teaspoons red wine 4 eggs 4 rashers of bacon, chopped 1 cup red onions, minced 1 teaspoon garlic, smashed 1 bay laurel 1 thyme sprig 1 rosemary sprig Kosher salt and black pepper, to taste

Directions Cook the bacon in a nonstick skillet over medium-high heat; reserve. Sauté the red onions and garlic in 1 tablespoon of bacon grease. Add in the cabbage and continue to cook, stirring frequently, until it has softened or about 4 minutes. Add a splash of wine to deglaze the pan. Add in the spices and continue to cook for a further 2 minutes. Fry the eggs in 1 tablespoon of bacon grease. Add in the reserved bacon and top with fried eggs.Bon appétit!

162.   Greek-Style Zucchini Patties

(Ready in about 15 minutes | Servings 6) Per serving: 153 Calories; 11.8g Fat; 6.6g Carbs; 6.4g Protein; 1.1g Fiber

Ingredients

1 pound zucchinis, shredded 1 cup Halloumi cheese, shredded 1/2 cup onion, finely chopped 1 teaspoon garlic, finely minced 2 tablespoons butter 1 egg, whisked 2 celery stalks, shredded 2 tablespoons cilantro, chopped Sea salt and pepper, to taste

Directions

Thoroughly combine all ingredients in a mixing bowl. Form the mixture into 12 patties and arrange them on a parchment-lined baking sheet. Bake in the preheated oven at 365 degrees F for 12 minutes, rotating the pan once or twice.Enjoy!

163.   Spicy Salad with Macadamia Nuts

(Ready in about 5 minutes | Servings 4) Per serving: 184 Calories; 16.8g Fat; 4g Carbs; 2.1g Protein; 1.4g Fiber

Ingredients

1 cup radishes, thinly sliced 2 cups butterhead lettuce, torn into bite-sized pieces 1 Lebanese cucumber, sliced 1 bell pepper, sliced 1 white onion, sliced 1 ounce macadamia nuts, chopped Sea salt, to season 1 tablespoon sunflower seeds 1/2 lemon, freshly squeezed 3 tablespoons olive oil 1/2 teaspoon Sriracha sauce

Directions

In a mixing bowl, toss all ingredients until well combined. Taste and adjust seasonings.

164.   Cream of Cauliflower Soup

(Ready in about 20 minutes | Servings 4) Per serving: 260 Calories; 22.5g Fat; 4.1g Carbs; 7.2g Protein; 4.2g Fiber

Ingredients

3 cups cauliflower, cut into florets 1 cup avocado, pitted and chopped Salt and pepper, to taste 1 thyme sprig 1 cup coconut milk, unsweetened 3 cups roasted vegetable broth

Directions In a heavy-bottomed pot, simmer the vegetable broth over medium-high heat. Add in the cauliflower and continue to simmer for 10 to 15 minutes more. Add in the coconut milk, avocado, salt, pepper, and thyme. Partially cover and continue to cook for a further 5 minutes. Puree the mixture in your blender.Enjoy!

165.   Greek-Style Vegetables

(Ready in about 15 minutes | Servings 4) Per serving: 318 Calories; 24.3g Fat; 5.1g Carbs; 15.4g Protein; 1.7g Fiber

Ingredients

1/2 pound brown mushrooms, chopped 1 cup broccoli, cut into small florets 1 medium-sized zucchini, chopped 8 ounces feta cheese, cubed 1 teaspoon Greek seasoning mix 2 tablespoons olive oil 1 onion, chopped 1 teaspoon garlic, minced 1 vine-ripened tomato, pureed 1/4 cup white wine

DirectionsIn a medium pot, heat the oil over a moderately-high heat. Sauté the onion and garlic for about 5 minutes, adding a splash of water if needed, until tender and aromatic. Add in the mushrooms, broccoli, zucchini, Greek seasoning mix, tomato puree, and white wine. Continue to cook for 4 to 5 minutes or until they've softened.Enjoy!

166.   Provençal-Style Green Beans

(Ready in about 15 minutes | Servings 4) Per serving: 183 Calories; 16.1g Fat; 4.4g Carbs; 3.2g Protein; 4g Fiber

Ingredients

1 pound green beans 1/2 teaspoon fresh garlic, minced 1/2 teaspoon red pepper flakes Salt and pepper, to taste 1 tablespoon butter, melted 1 celery stalk, shredded For Tapenade: 1 ½ tablespoons capers 2 anchovy fillets 1 tablespoon fresh lime juice 1/2 cup black olives 3 tablespoons extra-virgin olive oil

Directions

Steam the green beans approximately 4 minutes or until crisp-tender. In a saucepan, melt the butter over a moderately-high heat. Sauté the celery and garlic for 4 to 5 minutes or until they are tender and fragrant. Add in green beans and stir to combine. Season with red pepper, salt, and black pepper. To make the tapenade, pulse all ingredients until well combined.

167. Broccoli with Gruyère Cheese Sauce

(Ready in about 30 minutes | Servings 6) Per serving: 159 Calories; 12.3g Fat; 7.2g Carbs; 5.7g Protein; 5.5g Fiber

Ingredients

2 pounds broccoli, cut into small florets 1/4 teaspoon turmeric powder Sea salt and black pepper, to taste 1 ½ tablespoons olive oil 1/4 cup scallions, chopped 2 tablespoons green garlic, minced   For the Sauce: 1/3 cup sour cream 1/2 cup Gruyère cheese, shredded 1 ½ tablespoons butter

Directions

Parboil the broccoli florets in a large pot of boiling water for about 3 minutes until crisp-tender. Drain. Heat the oil in a frying pan over a moderately-high heat. Once hot, cook the scallions and green garlic for about 2 minutes or until tender and aromatic. Add in the curry turmeric powder, salt, pepper and continue to sauté for 3 minutes more or until aromatic. Add a splash of vegetable broth, partially cover, and continue to cook for 6 to 7 minutes. Add the reserved broccoli back to the pan. In another pan, melt the butter over a moderately-high heat. Add in the sour cream and cheese and stir over low heat for 2 to 3 minutes.Bon appétit!

168. Mushroom and Cauliflower Quiche

(Ready in about 35 minutes | Servings 4) Per serving: 275 Calories; 21.3g Fat; 5.3g Carbs; 14g Protein; 3g Fiber

Ingredients

1 pound cauliflower florets 1/2 pound brown mushrooms, thinly sliced 1 1/2 cup cream cheese 1 cup Gruyère cheese 1 cup cream of mushroom soup 1 teaspoon Italian herb mix 2 tablespoons butter 4 eggs, lightly beaten 1 teaspoon Dijon mustard

Directions

Melt the butter in a saucepan over medium-high heat. Now, cook the mushrooms until they release the liquid. Add in the cream of mushrooms soup, Italian herb mix, and cauliflower. Continue to sauté until the cauliflower has softened. Spoon the cauliflower mixture into a buttered casserole dish. In a mixing bowl, whisk the eggs, cheese, and Dijon mustard. Spoon the sauce over the top of your casserole. Bake in the preheated oven at 365 degrees F for about 30 minutes or until the top is hot and bubbly. Bon appétit!

169.   Japanese-Style Eringi Mushrooms

(Ready in about 15 minutes | Servings 3) Per serving: 103 Calories; 6.7g Fat; 5.9g Carbs; 2.7g Protein; 3.3g Fiber

Ingredients

8 ounces Eringi mushrooms, trim away about 1-inch of the root section Salt and Sansho pepper, to season 1 ½ tablespoons butter, melted 1 cup onions, finely chopped 2 cloves garlic, minced 2 tablespoons mirin 1/2 cup dashi stock 1 tablespoon lightly toasted sesame seeds

Directions

Melt the butter in a large pan over a moderately-high flame. Cook the onions and garlic for about 4 minutes, stirring continuously to ensure even cooking. Add in the Eringi mushrooms and continue to cook an additional 3 minutes until they are slightly shriveled. Season to taste and add in the mirin and dashi stock; continue to cook an additional 3 minutes.Enjoy!

170.   Artichoke Salad with Mozzarella Cheese

(Ready in about 25 minutes | Servings 6) Per serving: 146 Calories; 9.4g Fat; 6.1g Carbs; 5.8g Protein; 6g Fiber

Ingredients

2 tablespoons olive oil 3 artichoke hearts, defrosted Sea salt and black pepper, to taste 3/4 cup scallions, peeled and finely chopped 12/3 cup arugula   1/3 cup mustard greens 1/3 cup green cabbage 3 tablespoons capers, drained 1 chili pepper, sliced thin 3 teaspoon fresh lemon juice 1 ½ teaspoons deli mustard 2 tablespoons balsamic vinegar 2 tomatoes, sliced 2 ounces Kalamata olives, pitted and sliced 4 ounces Mozzarella cheese, crumbled

Directions

Start by preheating your oven to 350 degrees F. Line a baking sheet with parchment paper or a silicone mat. Brush the artickohe hearts with olive oil. Roast the artichoke hearts in the preheated oven at 360 degrees F for about 20 minutes. Season with salt and pepper to taste. Meanwhile, toss the vegetables with capers, lemon juice, mustard and balsamic vinegar until well combined.

171. Homemade Cold Gazpacho Soup

Ready in about: 15 minutes + chilling time | Serves: 6 Per serving: Kcal 528, Fat: 45.8g, Net Carbs: 6.5g, Protein: 7.5g

Ingredients

2 small green peppers, roasted 2 large red peppers, roasted 2 avocados, flesh scoped out 2 garlic cloves 2 spring onions, chopped 1 cucumber, chopped 1 cup olive oil 2 tbsp lemon juice 4 tomatoes, chopped 7 oz goat cheese, crumbled 1 small red onion, chopped 2 tbsp apple cider vinegar 1 tsp xylitol Salt to taste

Directions

Place the peppers, tomatoes, avocados, red onion, garlic, lemon juice, olive oil, vinegar, xylitol, and salt in a food processor. Pulse until your desired consistency is reached. Taste and adjust the seasoning. Transfer the mixture to a pot. Stir in cucumber and spring onions. Chill in the fridge for at least 2 hours. Divide the soup between 6 bowls. Serve topped with goat cheese and an extra drizzle of olive oil. Tip: For more protein, add cooked and chopped shrimp to this refreshing delight.

172. Power Green Soup

Ready in about: 30 minutes | Serves: 6 Per serving: Kcal 392, Fat: 37.6g, Net Carbs: 5.8g, Protein: 4.9g

Ingredients

1 broccoli head, chopped 1 cup spinach 1 onion, chopped 2 garlic cloves, minced ½ cup watercress 5 cups vegetable stock 1 cup coconut milk 1 tbsp ghee Salt and black pepper to taste

Directions

Melt the ghee in a large pot over medium heat. Add onion and garlic and cook for 3 minutes. Add broccoli and cook for an additional 5 minutes. Pour the vegetable stock over and close the lid. Bring to a boil. Reduce the heat. Simmer for 3 minutes. Add spinach and watercress and cook for 3 more minutes. Stir in the coconut cream, salt, and black pepper. Blend the soup with a hand blender. Serve warm.

173. Creamy Cauliflower Soup with Bacon Chips

Ready in about: 25 minutes | Serves: 4 Per serving: Kcal 402, Fat 37g, Net Carbs 6g, Protein 8g

Ingredients

2 tbsp ghee 1 onion, chopped 2 head cauliflower, cut into florets 2 cups water Salt and black pepper to taste 3 cups almond milk 1 cup white cheddar cheese, grated 3 bacon strips

Directions

Melt the ghee in a saucepan over medium heat and sauté the onion for 3 minutes until fragrant. Include the cauli florets and sauté for 3 minutes until slightly softened. Add the water and season with salt and black pepper. Bring to a boil and then reduce the heat. Cover and simme for 10 minutes. Puree the soup with an immersion blender until the ingredients are evenly Combined. Stir in the almond milk and cheese until the cheese Melts. In a non-stick skillet over high heat, fry the bacon for 5 minutes until crispy. Divide soup between serving bowls, top with crispy bacon, and serve hot.

174. Slow Cooker Beer Soup with Cheddar & Sausage

Ready in about: 8 hr | Serves: 6 Per serving: Kcal 244, Fat: 17g, Net Carbs: 4g, Protein: 5g

Ingredients

1 cup heavy cream 10 oz sausages, sliced 1 celery stalk, chopped 1 carrot, chopped 2 garlic cloves, minced 4 oz cream cheese, softened 1 tsp red pepper flakes 6 oz low carb beer 2 cups beef stock 1 onion, chopped 1 cup cheddar cheese, grated Salt and black pepper to taste

Directions

Turn on the slow cooker. Add in beef stock, beer, sausages, carrot, onion, garlic, celery, salt, red pepper flakes, and pepper and stir well. Pour in enough water to cover all the ingredients by roughly 2 inches. Close the lid and cook for 6 hours on Low. Open the lid and stir in the heavy cream, cheddar, and cream cheese and cook for 2 more hours. Ladle the soup into bowls and serve. Yummy!

175. Salsa Verde Chicken Soup

Ready in about: 15 minutes | Serves: 4 Per serving: Kcal 346, Fat: 23g, Net Carbs: 3g, Protein: 25g

Ingredients

½ cup salsa verde 2 cups cooked and shredded chicken 2 cups chicken broth 1 cup cheddar cheese, shredded 4 oz cream cheese, softened ½ tsp chili powder ½ tsp cumin 2 tsp fresh cilantro, chopped Salt and black pepper to taste

Directions

Combine the cream cheese, salsa verde, and broth in a food processor; pulse until smooth. Transfer the mixture to a pot and place over medium heat. Cook until hot, but do not bring to a boil. Add chicken, chili powder, and cumin and cook for about 3-5 minutes or until it is heated through. Stir in cheddar cheese and season with salt and pepper. If it is very thick, add a few tablespoons of water and boil for 1-3 more minutes. Serve hot in bowls sprinkled with fresh cilantro.

176. Thyme & Wild Mushroom Soup

Ready in about: 25 minutes | Serves: 4 Per serving: Kcal 281, Fat: 25g, Net Carbs: 5.8g, Protein: 6.1g

Ingredients

¼ cup butter ½ cup crème fraiche 12 oz wild mushrooms, chopped 2 tsp thyme leaves 2 garlic cloves, minced 4 cups chicken broth

DirectionsMelt the butter in a large pot over medium heat. Add garlic and cook for 1 minute until tender. Add mushrooms and cook for 10 minutes. Pour in the broth over and bring to a boil. Simmer for 10 minutes. Puree the soup with a hand blender until smooth. Stir in crème fraiche. Garnish with thyme to serve.

177. Brazilian Moqueca (Shrimp Stew)

Ready in about: 25 minutes | Serves: 6 Per serving: Kcal 324, Fat: 21g, Net Carbs: 5g, Protein: 23.1g

Ingredients 1 cup coconut milk 2 tbsp lime juice ¼ cup diced roasted peppers 1 ½ lb shrimp, peeled and deveined ¼ cup olive oil 1 garlic clove, minced 14 oz diced tomatoes 2 tbsp sriracha sauce 1 onion, chopped ¼ cup chopped cilantro 2 tbsp fresh dill, chopped to garnish Salt and black pepper to taste

DirectionsHeat the olive oil in a pot over medium heat. Add onion and garlic and cook for 3 minutes until translucent. Stir in tomatoes, shrimp, and cilantro. Cook until the shrimp becomes opaque, about 3-4 minutes. Pour in sriracha sauce and coconut milk, and cook for 2 minutes. Do not bring to a boil. Stir in the lime juice and season with salt and pepper. Spoon the stew in bowls, garnish with fresh dill, and serve.

178.   Cobb Egg Salad in Lettuce Cups

Ready in about: 25 minutes | Serves: 4 Per serving: Kcal 325, Fat 24.5g, Net Carbs 4g, Protein 21g

Ingredients

1 head green lettuce, firm leaves removed for cups 2 chicken breasts, cut into pieces 1 tbsp olive oil Salt and black pepper to taste 6 large eggs 2 tomatoes, seeded, chopped 6 tbsp Greek yogurt Preheat oven to 400°F.

Directions

Put the chicken in a bowl, drizzle with olive oil, and sprinkle with salt and black pepper. Toss to coat. Put the chicken on a baking sheet and spread out evenly. Slide the baking sheet in the oven and bake the chicken until cooked through and golden brown for 8 minutes, stirring once. Boil the eggs in salted water for 10 minutes. Let them cool, peel, and chop into pieces. Transfer to a salad bowl. Remove the chicken from the oven and add to the salad bowl. Include the tomatoes and Greek yogurt and mix them. Layer 2 lettuce leaves each as cups and fill with 2 tbsp of egg salad each. Serve.

179.   Arugula Prawn Salad with Mayo Dressing

Ready in about: 15 minutes | Serves: 4 Per serving: Kcal 215, Fat 20.3g, Net Carbs 2g, Protein 8g

Ingredients

4 cups baby arugula ½ cup mayonnaise 3 tbsp olive oil 1 lb prawns, peeled and deveined 1 tsp Dijon mustard Salt to taste ½ tsp chili pepper 2 tbsp lemon juice ½ tsp garlic powder

DirectionsMix the mayonnaise, lemon juice, garlic, powder, and mustard in a small bowl until smooth and creamy. Set aside until ready to use. Heat 2 tbsp of olive oil in a skillet over medium heat. Add the prawns, season with salt and chili pepper, and fry for 3 minutes on each side until prawns are pink. Set aside to a plate. Place the arugula in a serving bowl and pour the mayo dressing over the salad. Toss with 2 spoons until mixed. Divide the salad between 4 plates and top with prawns. Serve immediately.

180.   Mozzarella & Tomato Salad with Anchovies & Olives

Ready in about: 10 minutes | Serves: 2 Per serving: Kcal 430, Fat: 26.8g, Net Carbs: 2.4g, Protein:38.8g

Ingredients 1 large tomato, sliced 4 basil leaves 8 mozzarella cheese slices 2 tsp olive oil 2 canned anchovies, chopped 1 tsp balsamic vinegar 4 black olives, pitted and sliced Salt to taste

DirectionsArrange the tomato slices on a serving plate. Place the mozzarella slices over and top with the basil. Add the anchovies and olives on top. Drizzle with olive oil and vinegar. Sprinkle with salt and serve.

181. Spring Salad with Cheese Balls

Ready in about: 20 minutes | Serves: 6 Per serving: Kcal: 234; Fat 16.7g, Net Carbs 7.9g, Protein 12.4g

Ingredients

Cheese balls 3 eggs 1 cup feta cheese, crumbled ½ cup Pecorino cheese, shredded 1 cup almond flour 1 tbsp flax meal Salt and black pepper to taste Salad 1 head Iceberg lettuce, leaves separated ½ cup cucumber, thinly sliced 2 tomatoes, seeded and chopped ½ cup red onion, thinly sliced ½ cup radishes, thinly sliced ⅓ cup mayonnaise 1 tsp mustard 1 tsp paprika 1 tsp oregano Salt to taste Preheat oven to 390°F.

Directions

In a mixing dish, mix all ingredients for the cheese balls. Form balls out of the mixture. Set the balls on a lined baking sheet. Bake for 10 minutes until crisp. Arrange lettuce leaves on a large salad platter. Add in radishes, tomatoes, cucumbers, and red onion. In a small mixing bowl, mix the mayonnaise, paprika, salt, oregano, and mustard. Sprinkle the mixture over the vegetables. Add cheese balls on top and serve.

182. Shrimp & Avocado Cauliflower Salad

Ready in about: 30 minutes | Serves: 6 Per serving: Kcal 214, Fat: 17g, Net Carbs: 5g, Protein: 15g

Ingredients

1 cauliflower head, florets only 1 lb medium shrimp, peeled ¼ cup + 1 tbsp olive oil 1 avocado, chopped 2 tbsp fresh dill, chopped ¼ cup lemon juice 2 tbsp lemon zest Salt and black pepper to taste

Directions

Heat 1 tbsp olive oil in a skillet and cook shrimp for 8 minutes. Microwave cauliflower for 5 minutes. Place shrimp, cauliflower, and avocado in a bowl. Whisk the remaining olive oil, lemon zest, juice, dill, and salt, and pepper in another bowl. Pour the dressing over, toss to Combine, and serve immediately.

183.   Bacon & Spinach Salad

Ready in about: 20 minutes | Serves: 4 Per serving: Kcal 350, Fat: 33g, Net Carbs: 3.4g, Protein: 7g

Ingredients

1 avocado, chopped 1 avocado, sliced 1 spring onion, sliced 4 bacon slices, chopped 2 cups spinach 2 small lettuce heads, chopped 2 eggs 3 tbsp olive oil 1 tsp Dijon mustard 1 tbsp apple cider vinegar Salt to taste

Directions

Place a skillet over medium heat and cook the bacon for 5 minutes until crispy. Remove to paper-towel lined plate to drain. Boil the eggs in boiling salted water for 10 minutes. Let them cool, peel, and chop. Combine the spinach, lettuce, eggs, chopped avocado, and spring onion in a large bowl. Whisk together the olive oil, mustard, apple cider vinegar, and salt in another bowl. Pour the dressing over the salad and toss to Combine. Top with the sliced avocado and bacon and serve.

184.   Italian-Style Green Salad

Ready in about: 15 minutes | Serves: 4 Per serving: Kcal 205, Fat 20g, Net Carbs 2g, Protein 4g

Ingredients

2 (8 oz) pack mixed salad greens 8 pancetta strips 1 cup gorgonzola cheese, crumbled 1 tbsp white wine vinegar 3 tbsp extra virgin olive oil Salt and black pepper to taste

Directions

Fry the pancetta strips in a skillet over medium heat for 6 minutes, until browned and crispy. Remove to paper-towel lined plate to drain. Chop it when it is cooled. Pour the salad greens into a serving bowl. In a small bowl, whisk the white wine vinegar, olive oil, salt, and pepper. Drizzle the dressing over the salad and toss to coat. Top with gorgonzola cheese and pancetta. Divide salad into plates and serve.

185. Warm Baby Artichoke Salad

Ready in about: 30 minutes | Serves: 4 Per serving: Kcal 170, Fat: 13g, Net Carbs: 5g, Protein: 1g

Ingredients

6 baby artichokes 6 cups water 1 tbsp lemon juice ¼ cup cherry peppers, halved ¼ cup pitted olives, sliced ¼ cup olive oil ¼ tsp lemon zest 2 tsp balsamic vinegar, sugar-free 1 tbsp chopped dill Salt and black pepper to taste 1 tbsp capers ¼ tsp caper brine

Directions

Combine the water and salt in a pot over medium heat. Trim and halve the artichokes. Add them to the pot and bring to a boil. Lower the heat and let simmer for 20 minutes until tender. Combine the rest of the ingredients, except for the olives, in a bowl. Drain and place the artichokes on a serving plate. Pour the prepared mixture over; toss to Combine well. Serve topped with the olives.

186. Spinach & Turnip Salad with Bacon

Ready in about: 40 minutes | Serves: 4 Per serving: Kcal 193, Fat 18.3g, Net Carbs 3.1g, Protein 9.5g

Ingredients

2 turnips, cut into wedges 1 tsp olive oil 1 cup baby spinach, chopped 3 radishes, sliced 3 turkey bacon slices 4 tbsp sour cream 2 tsp mustard seeds 1 tsp Dijon mustard 1 tbsp red wine vinegar Salt and black pepper to taste 1 tbsp chopped chives Preheat oven to 400°F.

Directions

Line a baking sheet with parchment paper, toss the turnips with salt and black pepper, drizzle with the olive oil, and bake for 25 minutes, turning halfway. Let cool. Spread the baby spinach in the bottom of a salad bowl and top with the radishes. Remove the turnips to the salad bowl. Fry the bacon in a skillet over medium heat until crispy, about 5 minutes. Mix sour cream, mustard seeds, mustard, vinegar, and salt with the bacon. Add a little water to deglaze the bottom of the skillet. Pour the bacon mixture over the vegetables, scatter the chives over it. Serve.

187. Cobb Salad with Blue Cheese Dressing

Ready in about: 30 minutes | Serves: 6 Per serving: Kcal 122, Fat 14g, Net Carbs 2g, Protein 23g

Ingredients

Dressing ½ cup buttermilk 1 cup mayonnaise 2 tbsp Worcestershire sauce ½ cup sour cream 1 cup blue cheese, crumbled 2 tbsp chives, chopped Salad 6 eggs 2 chicken breasts 5 strips bacon 1 iceberg lettuce, cut into chunks Salt and black pepper to taste 1 romaine lettuce, chopped 1 bibb lettuce, cored, leaves removed 2 avocado, pitted and diced 2 large tomatoes, chopped ½ cup blue cheese, crumbled 2 scallions, chopped

DirectionsIn a bowl, whisk the buttermilk, mayonnaise, Worcestershire sauce, and sour cream. Stir in the blue cheese and chives. Place in the refrigerator to chill until ready to use. Bring the eggs to boil in salted water over medium heat for 10 minutes. Transfer to an ice bath to cool. Peel and chop. Set aside. Preheat a grill pan over high heat. Season the chicken with salt and pepper. Grill for 3 minutes on each side. Remove to a plate to cool for 3 minutes and cut into bite-size chunks. Fry the bacon in the same pan until crispy, about 6 minutes. Remove, let cool for 2 minutes, and chop. Arrange the lettuce leaves in a salad bowl, and in single piles, add the avocado, tomatoes, eggs, bacon, and chicken. Sprinkle the blue cheese over the salad as well as the scallions and black pepper. Drizzle the blue cheese dressing on the salad and serve with low carb bread.

188. Pancetta and Goat Cheese-Stuffed Mushrooms

(Ready in about 25 minutes | Servings 6) Per serving: 98 Calories; 5.8g Fat; 3.9g Carbs; 8.4g Protein; 0.6g Fiber

Ingredients

12 medium-sized button mushrooms, stems removed 3 slices of pancetta, chopped 2 ounces goat cheese, crumbled 2 tablespoons butter, melted 1 tablespoon oyster sauce Sea salt and black pepper, to taste 1 teaspoon basil 1 teaspoon fresh rosemary, minced

Directions

Brush your mushrooms with melted butter and oyster sauce. Season them with salt and pepper to taste. Mix the pancetta, basil, rosemary, and goat cheese. Spoon the mixture into the mushroom caps and arrange them on a parchment-lined baking sheet. Bake in the preheated oven at 360 degrees F for about 20 minutes or until tender.Enjoy!

189. Roasted Autumn Vegetables

(Ready in about 35 minutes | Servings 6) Per serving: 137 Calories; 11.1g Fat; 3.1g Carbs; 1.2g Protein; 2.3g Fiber

Ingredients

3 tablespoons olive oil 1 onion, cut into wedges 1 fresh chili pepper, minced 1/2 pound celery, quartered 1/2 pound bell peppers, sliced 1/2 pound turnips, cut into wedges Sea salt and ground black pepper, to taste 1 teaspoon dried thyme 1 teaspoon dried basil 1 garlic clove, minced

Directions

Toss all ingredients in a roasting pan. Roast in the preheated oven at 410 degrees F for 30 minutes. Taste and adjust the seasoning.Bon appétit!

190. Grilled Zucchini with Mediterranean Sauce

(Ready in about 15 minutes | Servings 4) Per serving: 132 Calories; 11.1g Fat; 4.1g Carbs; 3.1g Protein; 1.3g Fiber

Ingredients

1 pound zucchini, cut lengthwise into quarters 1/2 teaspoon red pepper flakes, crushed Salt, to season 1/4 cup extra-virgin olive oil 1 teaspoon garlic, minced For the Sauce: 1 tablespoon fresh scallions, minced 1 tablespoon fresh basil, chopped 1 teaspoon fresh rosemary, finely chopped 3/4 cup Greek-style yogurt

Directions

Begin by preheating your grill to a medium-low heat. Toss the zucchini slices with the olive oil, garlic, red pepper, and salt. Grill your zucchini on a lightly-oiled grill for about 10 minutes until tender and slightly charred. Make the sauce by whisking all of the sauce ingredients.Enjoy!

191.Autumn Eggplant and Squash Stew

(Ready in about 35 minutes | Servings 6) Per serving: 113 Calories; 7.9g Fat; 3.7g Carbs; 2.8g Protein; 2.2g Fiber

Ingredients

2 tablespoons olive 2 garlic cloves, finely chopped 3 ounces acorn squash, chopped 1 celery, chopped 2 tablespoons fresh parsley, roughly chopped Sea salt and pepper, to taste 1/2 teaspoon ancho chili powder 2 tomatoes, pureed 2 tablespoons port wine 1 large onion, chopped 3 ounces eggplant, peeled and chopped

Directions

In a heavy-bottomed pot, heat olive oil over a moderately-high heat. Sauté the onion and garlic about 5 minutes. Add in the acorn squash, eggplant, celery and parsley; continue to cook for 5 to 6 minutes. Add in the other ingredients; turn the heat to a simmer. Continue to cook for about 25 minutes.Enjoy!

192.   Cheesy Italian Pepper Casserole

(Ready in about 1 hour | Servings 4) Per serving: 408 Calories; 28.9g Fat; 4.6g Carbs; 24.9g Protein; 3.5g Fiber

Ingredients

8 Italian sweet peppers, deveined and cut into fourths lengthwise 6 whole eggs 1/2 cup Greek-style yogurt 3/4 pound Asiago cheese, shredded 1 leek, thinly sliced 1/2 teaspoon garlic, crushed Sea salt and ground black pepper, to taste 1 teaspoon oregano

Directions Arrange the peppers in a lightly greased baking dish. Top with half of the shredded cheese; add a layer of sliced leeks and garlic. Repeat the layers. After that, beat the eggs with the yogurt, salt, pepper, and oregano. Pour the egg/yogurt mixture over the peppers. Cover with a piece of foil and bake for about 30 minutes. Remove the foil and bake for a further 10 to 15 minutes.Bon appétit!

193.   Easy Vegetable Ratatouille

(Ready in about 1 hour | Servings 4) Per serving: 159 Calories; 10.4g Fat; 5.7g Carbs; 6.4g Protein; 5g Fiber

Ingredients 1 large onion, sliced 1/3 cup Parmesan cheese, shredded 1 celery, peeled and diced 1 poblano pepper, minced 1 eggplant, cut into thick slices 1 cup grape tomatoes, halved 1/2 garlic head, minced 2 tablespoons extra-virgin olive oil 1 tablespoon fresh basil leaves, snipped

Directions Sprinkle the eggplant with 1 teaspoon of salt and let it stand for about 30 minutes; drain and rinse under running water. Place the eggplant slices in the bottom of a lightly-oiled casserole dish. Add in the remaining vegetable. Add in the olive oil and basil leaves. Bake in the preheated oven at 350 degrees F for about 30 minute or until thoroughly cooked.Bon appétit!

194. Spring Mixed Greens Salad

(Ready in about 10 minutes | Servings 4) Per serving: 190 Calories; 17.6g Fat; 7.6g Carbs; 4.3g Protein; 3.9g Fiber

Ingredients

1 cup romaine lettuce 1 cup lollo rosso 1/3 cup goat cheese, crumbled 2 tablespoons fresh parsley, chopped 2 tablespoons extra-virgin olive oil 1/2 lime, freshly squeezed 2 cups baby spinach 1/2 cup blueberries 1 cup avocado, pitted, peeled and sliced Sea salt and white pepper, to taste

Directions

Toss all ingredients in a mixing bowl. Taste and adjust seasonings. Place in your refrigerator until ready to use.

195. Cream of Thyme Tomato Soup

Ready in about: 20 minutes | Serves: 4 Per serving: Kcal 310, Fat 27g, Net Carbs 3g, Protein 11g

Ingredients

2 tbsp ghee 2 large red onions, diced ½ cup raw cashew nuts, diced 2 (28 oz) cans tomatoes 2 tsp fresh thyme leaves 1 ½ cups water Salt and black pepper to taste 1 cup heavy cream

Directions

Melt ghee in a pot over medium heat and sauté the onions for 4 minutes until softened. Stir in the tomatoes, thyme, water, and cashews and season with salt and black pepper. Cover and bring to a boil. Simmer for 10 minutes until thoroughly cooked. Open, turn the heat off, and puree the ingredients with an immersion blender. Adjust the taste and stir in the heavy cream. Spoon into soup bowls and serve.

196. Green Minestrone Soup

Ready in about: 25 minutes | Serves: 4 Per serving: Kcal 227, Fat 20.3g, Net Carbs 2g, Protein 8g

Ingredients 2 tbsp ghee 2 tbsp onion-garlic puree 2 heads broccoli, cut into florets 2 celery stalks, chopped 4 cups vegetable broth 1 cup baby spinach Salt and black pepper to taste 2 tbsp Gruyere cheese, grated

DirectionsMelt the ghee in a saucepan over medium heat and sauté the onion-garlic puree for 3 minutes until softened. Mix in the broccoli and celery, and cook for 4 minutes until slightly tender. Pour in the broth, bring to a boil, then reduce the heat to medium-low and simmer covered for about 5 minutes. Drop in the spinach to wilt, adjust the seasonings, and cook for 4 minutes. Ladle soup into serving bowls. Serve with a sprinkle of grated Gruyere cheese.

197. Buffalo Chicken Soup

Ready in about: 40 minutes | Serves: 4 Per serving: Kcal 215, Fat: 11.3g, Net Carbs: 2.4g, Protein: 7.5g

Ingredients

2 chicken legs 2 tbsp butter, melted 1 onion, chopped 2 garlic cloves, minced 1 carrot, chopped 1 bay leaf 2 tbsp fresh cilantro, chopped ⅓ cup buffalo sauce Salt and black pepper to taste

Directions

Add the chicken in a pot over medium heat and cover with water. Add in salt, pepper, and bay leaf. Boil for 15 minutes. Remove to a plate and let it cool slightly. Strain and reserve the broth. Melt the butter in a large saucepan over medium heat. Sauté the onion, garlic, and carrot for 5 minutes until tender, stirring occasionally. Remove skin and bones from chicken and discard. Chop the chicken and add it to the saucepan. Stir in the buffalo sauce for 1 minute and pour in the broth. Bring to a boil. Cook for 15 minutes. Adjust the taste with salt and pepper and top with cilantro. Serve.

198. Coconut Green Bean & Shrimp Curry Soup

Ready in about: 20 minutes | Serves: 4 Per serving: Kcal 375, Fat 35.4g, Net Carbs 2g, Protein 9g

Ingredients

1 lb jumbo shrimp, peeled and deveined 2 tbsp ghee 2 tsp ginger-garlic puree 2 tbsp red curry paste 6 oz coconut milk Salt and chili pepper to taste 1 lb green beans, trimmed, chopped

Directions

Melt the ghee in a medium saucepan over medium heat. Add the shrimp, season with salt and black pepper, and cook until opaque, about 2-3 minutes. Remove the shrimp to a plate. Add the ginger-garlic puree and red curry paste to the ghee and sauté for 2 more minutes until fragrant. Stir in the coconut milk. Add in the shrimp, salt, chili pepper, and green beans. Cook for 4 minutes. Reduce the heat to a simmer and cook for an additional 5-7 minutes, occasionally stirring. Adjust the taste with salt and fetch soup into serving bowls. Serve with cauli rice.

199. Creamy Cauliflower Soup with Chorizo Sausage

Ready in about: 40 minutes | Serves: 4 Per serving: Kcal 251, Fat: 19.1g, Net Carbs: 5.7g, Protein: 10g

Ingredients

1 cauliflower head, chopped 1 turnip, chopped 3 tbsp butter 1 chorizo sausage, sliced 2 cups chicken broth 1 small onion, chopped 2 cups water Salt and black pepper to taste

Directions

Melt 2 tbsp of the butter in a large pot over medium heat. Stir in the onion and cook until soft, 3-4 minutes. Add cauliflower and turnip and cook for another 5 minutes. Pour the broth and water over. Bring to a boil. Simmer covered for about 20 minutes until the vegetables are tender. Remove from heat. Melt the remaining butter in a skillet. Cook the chorizo for 5 minutes until crispy. Puree the soup with a hand blender until smooth. Adjust the seasonings. Serve the soup topped with the chorizo sausage.

200. Pumpkin & Meat Peanut Stew

Ready in about: 45 minutes | Serves: 6 Per serving: Kcal 451, Fat: 33g, Net Carbs: 4g, Protein: 27.5g

Ingredients 1 cup pumpkin puree 2 lb chopped pork stew meat 1 tbsp peanut butter 4 tbsp peanuts, chopped 1 garlic clove, minced 1 onion, chopped ½ cup white wine 1 tbsp olive oil 1 tsp lemon juice ¼ cup granulated sweetener ¼ tsp cardamom powder ¼ tsp allspice 2 cups water 2 cups chicken stock

DirectionsHeat the olive oil in a large pot and sauté onion and garlic for 3 minutes until translucent. Add the pork and brown for about 5-6 minutes, stirring occasionally. Pour in the wine and cook for 1 minute. Add in the remaining ingredients, except for the lemon juice and peanuts. Bring the mixture to a boil and cook for 5 minutes. Reduce the heat to low, cover the pot, and let cook for about 30 minutes. Adjust seasonings and stir in the lemon juice before serving. Ladle into bowls and serve topped with peanuts.

201. Mediterranean Salad

Ready in about: 10 minutes | Serves: 4 Per serving: Kcal 290, Fat: 25g, Net Carbs: 4.3g, Protein: 9g

Ingredients

3 tomatoes, sliced 1 large avocado, sliced 8 kalamata olives ¼ lb buffalo mozzarella, sliced 2 tbsp pesto sauce 1 tbsp olive oil

DirectionsArrange the tomato slices on a serving platter and place the avocado slices in the middle. Arrange the olives around the avocado slices and drop pieces of the mozzarella cheese on the platter. Drizzle the pesto sauce and olive oil all over and serve.

202.   Blue Cheese Chicken Salad

Ready in about: 15 minutes | Serves: 4 Per serving: Kcal 286, Fat 23g, Net Carbs 4g, Protein 14g

Ingredients

1 chicken breast, flattened Salt and black pepper to taste 4 tbsp olive oil 1 lb spinach and spring mix 1 tbsp red wine vinegar 1 cup blue cheese, crumbled

DirectionsSeason the chicken with salt and black pepper. Heat half of the olive oil in a pan over medium heat and fry the chicken for 4 minutes on both sides until golden brown. Remove and let cool before slicing. In a salad bowl, Combine the spinach and spring mix with the remaining olive oil, red wine vinegar, and salt and mix well. Top the salad with the chicken slices and sprinkle with blue cheese. Serve.

203.   Lobster Salad with Salsa Rosa

Ready in about: 10 minutes | Serves: 4 Per serving: Kcal 256, Fat: 15g, Net Carbs: 4.3g, Protein: 17.9g

Ingredients

2 hard-boiled eggs, sliced 1 cucumber, peeled and chopped ½ cup black olives 2 cups cooked lobster meat, diced 1 head Iceberg lettuce, shredded ½ cup mayonnaise ¼ tsp celery seeds Salt to taste 2 tbsp lemon juice ½ tsp sugar-free ketchup ¼ tsp dark rum

Directions

Combine the lettuce, cucumber, and lobster meat in a large bowl. Whisk together the mayonnaise, celery seeds, ketchup, rum, salt, and lemon juice in another bowl. Pour the dressing over the salad and gently toss to Combine. Top with olives and sliced eggs and serve.

204.   Strawberry Salad with Cheese & Almonds

Ready in about: 20 minutes | Serves: 2 Per serving: Kcal 445, Fat: 34.2g, Net Carbs: 5.3g, Protein: 33g

Ingredients

4 cups kale, chopped 4 strawberries, sliced ½ cup almonds, flaked 1 ½ cups hard goat cheese, grated 4 tbsp raspberry vinaigrette Salt and black pepper to taste Preheat oven to 400°F.

DirectionsArrange the grated goat cheese in two circles on two pieces of parchment paper. Place in the oven and bake for 10 minutes. Find two same bowls, place them upside down, and carefully put the parchment paper on top to give the cheese a bowl-like shape. Let cool that way for 15 minutes. Divide the kale among the bowls, sprinkle with salt and pepper and drizzle with vinaigrette. Toss to coat. Top with almonds and strawberries. Serve immediately.

205.   Green Mackerel Salad

Ready in about: 25 minutes | Serves: 4 Per serving: Kcal 356, Fat: 31.9g, Net Carbs: 0.8g, Protein: 1.3g

Ingredients

4 oz smoked mackerel, flaked 2 eggs 1 tbsp coconut oil 1 cup green beans, chopped 1 avocado, sliced 4 cups mixed salad greens 2 tbsp olive oil 1 tbsp lemon juice Salt and black pepper to taste .

Directions

In a bowl, whisk together the lemon juice, olive oil, salt, and pepper. Set aside. Cook the green beans in boiling salted water over medium heat for about 3 minutes. Remove with a slotted spoon and let to cool. Add the eggs to the pot and cook for 8-10 minutes. Transfer the eggs to an ice water bath, peel the shells, and slice them. Place the mixed salad green in a serving bowl and add in the green beans and smoked mackerel. Pour the dressing over and toss to coat. Top with sliced eggs and avocado and serve.

206.   Caesar Salad with Smoked Salmon & Poached Eggs

Ready in about: 15 minutes | Serves: 4 Per serving: Kcal 260, Fat 21g, Net Carbs 5g, Protein 8g

Ingredients

8 eggs 2 cups torn romaine lettuce ½ cup smoked salmon, chopped 6 slices bacon 2 tbsp low carb Caesar dressing 1 tbsp white wine vinegar

Directions

Bring a pot of water to a boil and pour in the vinegar. Crack each egg into a small bowl and gently slide into the water. Poach for 2 to 3 minutes, remove with a perforated spoon, and transfer to a paper towel to remove any excess water, and plate. Poach the remaining 7 eggs. Put the bacon in a skillet and fry over medium heat until browned and crispy, about 6 minutes, turning once. Remove, allow cooling, and chop into small pieces. Toss the lettuce, smoked salmon, bacon, and Caesar dressing in a salad bowl. Top with two eggs each and serve immediately or chilled.

DESSERT

207. Mini Brownies with Almonds

(Ready in about 25 minutes | Servings 12) Per serving: 251 Calories; 21.5g Fat; 4.6g Carbs; 6.4g Protein; 0.8g Fiber

Ingredients

4 ounces cocoa powder 1/2 cup almonds, ground 5 eggs 1/2 teaspoon ground cinnamon 6 ounces sour cream 2 tablespoons Swerve 2/3 cup coconut oil, melted 1 teaspoon rum extract 3/4 teaspoon baking powder

Directions

Begin by preheating your oven to 365 degrees F. Brush a muffin tin with a nonstick spray. Mix all ingredients in a bowl and scrape the batter into the muffin cups. Bake for about 20 minutes; let it cool slightly before unmolding and storing.Enjoy!

208. Rum Chocolate Pralines

(Ready in about 10 minutes + chilling time | Servings 8) Per serving: 70 Calories; 3.4g Fat; 5.1g Carbs; 2.4g Protein; 1.6g Fiber

Ingredients 1 cup bakers' chocolate, sugar-free 2 tablespoons dark rum 1/8 teaspoon ground cloves 1/8 teaspoon cinnamon powder 1/2 teaspoon almond extract 1/2 teaspoon rum extract 3 tablespoons cocoa powder 1/4 cup almond butter 1 cup almond milk

Directions

Microwave the chocolate, cocoa and almond butter until they have completely melted. Add in the other ingredients and mix to combine well. Pour the mixture into silicone molds and place in your refrigerator until set. Bon appétit!

209. Vanilla Berry Meringues

(Ready in about 2 hours | Servings 10) Per serving: 51 Calories; 0g Fat; 4g Carbs; 12g Protein; 0.1g Fiber

Ingredients 1 teaspoon vanilla extract 3 tablespoons freeze-dried mixed berries, crushed 3 large egg whites, at room temperature 1/3 cup Erythritol 1 teaspoon lemon rind

Directions In a mixing bowl, beat the egg whites until foamy. Add in vanilla extract, lemon rind, and Erythritol; continue to mix, using an electric mixer until stiff and glossy. Add the crushed berries and mix again until well combined. Use two teaspoons to spoon meringue onto parchment-lined cookie sheets. Bake at 220 degrees F for about 1 hour 45 minutes.Bon appétit!

210.   Mother's Day Pecan Truffles

(Ready in about 25 minutes + chilling time | Servings 6) Per serving: 113 Calories; 8.5g Fat; 5.9g Carbs; 1.7g Protein; 3.3g Fiber

Ingredients

1/2 cup toasted pecans, finely chopped 1/2 cup double cream 1 teaspoon vanilla paste 3 bars chocolate, sugar-free 1/4 teaspoon ground cardamom 1/4 teaspoon ground cinnamon 1/4 teaspoon coarse salt

Directions

In a medium stainless steel bowl set over a pot of gently simmering water, melt the chocolate and cream. Add in the vanilla, cardamom, cinnamon, and salt and place in your refrigerator for 7 to 8 hours or until firm. Shape the mixture into balls and roll the balls into the chopped pecans.Bon appétit!

211.Blueberry and Coconut Protein Shake

(Ready in about 10 minutes | Servings 4) Per serving: 274 Calories; 26.8g Fat; 7.5g Carbs; 3.9g Protein; 1.3g Fiber

Ingredients 1/2 cup blueberries, frozen 1/2 teaspoon vanilla essence 1/2 teaspoon Monk fruit powder 2 tablespoons collagen protein 2 tablespoons coconut cream 1/4 cup coconut shreds 1 cup coconut milk

Directions

Pulse the frozen blueberries in your blender. Add in the other ingredients and mix until creamy, smooth and uniform.

212.   Classic Chocolate Bars

(Ready in about 25 minutes + chilling time | Servings 10) Per serving: 119 Calories; 11.7g Fat; 5.2g Carbs; 1.1g Protein; 5g Fiber

Ingredients 1/2 stick butter, cold 1 ½ cups whipped cream A pinch of coarse salt 8 ounces chocolate chunks, sugar-free 1/4 teaspoon cinnamon 1/2 teaspoon rum extract 1 teaspoon vanilla extract 1/4 cup coconut flour 1/4 cup flaxseed meal 1 cup almond meal 2 packets stevia

Directions Start by preheating your oven to 340 degrees F. Coat a baking dish with a piece of parchment paper. Add the coconut flour, flaxseed meal, almond meal, stevia, cinnamon, rum extract, vanilla, and salt to your blender. Blend until everything is well incorporated. Cut in the cold butter and continue to blend until well combined. Spoon the batter into the bottom of the prepared baking pan. Bake for 12 to 15 minutes and place on a wire rack to cool slightly. Bring the whipped cream to a simmer; add in the chocolate chunks and whisk to combine. Spread the chocolate filling over the crust and place in your refrigerator until set. Cut into bars.Bon appétit!

213.   The Best Chocolate Cake Ever

(Ready in about 50 minutes + chilling time | Servings 10) Per serving: 313 Calories; 30.7g Fat; 7.5g Carbs; 7.3g Protein; 1.9g Fiber

Ingredients

5 eggs 1/2 teaspoon ground cinnamon A pinch of coarse salt 1/2 cup water 3/4 cup erythritol 14 ounces chocolate, unsweetened 2 sticks butter, cold

For Peanut-Choc Ganache:

9 ounces chocolate, unsweetened 1/4 cup smooth peanut butter A pinch of coarse salt 3/4 cups whipped cream

Directions

In a medium-sized pan, bring the water to a boil; add in the erythritol and let it simmer until it has dissolved. Melt the chocolate and butter; beat the mixture with an electric mixer. Add the chocolate mixture to the hot water mixture. Fold in the eggs, one at a time, beating continuously. Add in the cinnamon and salt, and stir well to combine. Spoon the mixture into a parchment-lined baking pan and wrap with foil. Lower the baking pan into a larger pan that is filled with hot water about 1 inch deep. Bake in the preheated oven at 365 degrees F for about 45 minutes. Meanwhile, place the whipped cream in a pan over a moderately-high heat and bring to a boil. Pour the hot cream over the chocolate and whisk to combine. Add in the peanut butter and salt; continue to mix until creamy and smooth. Glaze your cake and place in the refrigerator until set.Enjoy!

214.   Creamsicle Pudding with Coconut

(Ready in about 1 hour 5 minutes | Servings 4) Per serving: 226 Calories; 17.9g Fat; 7g Carbs; 5.9g Protein; 4.6g Fiber

Ingredients

1 cup unsweetened coconut milk 1 cup water 1/4 cup coconut flakes 2 tablespoons Swerve 1/2 teaspoon ground star anise 1 cup double cream 1 teaspoon coconut extract 1 cup chia seeds

Directions

Mix the ingredients until everything is well incorporated. Place in your refrigerator for about 1 hour.Enjoy!

215. Father's Day Ice Cream

(Ready in about 15 minutes + chilling time | Servings 8) Per serving: 89 Calories; 9.3g Fat; 1.5g Carbs; 0.8g Protein; 0g Fiber

Ingredients

3/4 cup double cream 1/2 cup coconut milk 1 tablespoon rum flavoring 24 packets of stevia A pinch of grated nutmeg A pinch of salt 1/4 cup Greek-style yogurt

Directions

Melt the double cream and coconut milk in a saucepan over a medium-low heat. Stir until there are no lumps. Allow it to cool and add in the other ingredients. Beat the ingredients using an electric mixer until creamy and uniform.Bon appétit!

216. Classic Chocolate Fudge

(Ready in about 15 minutes + chilling time | Servings 8) Per serving: 220 Calories; 20g Fat; 7g Carbs; 1.7g Protein; 2.1g Fiber

Ingredients

3/4 cup chocolate chunks, unsweetened 2 tablespoons coconut oil 4-5 drops Monk fruit sweetener 1/2 cup double cream 1/2 cup butter, at room temperature 1 cup full-fat milk

Directions

Microwave the chocolate and milk until they've completely melted; spoon into a foil-lined pie pan and freeze until firm. Then, melt the butter, coconut oil, Monk fruit sweetener, and double cream; mix with a wire whisk to combine well. Spoon the cream mixture over the chocolate layer and freeze until solid.Enjoy!

217.Butterscotch Pudding Popsicles

(Ready in about 1 hour | Servings 6) Per serving: 248 Calories; 20.8g Fat; 7g Carbs; 4.6g Protein; 4.1g Fiber

Ingredients

1 teaspoon orange juice 1 cup buttermilk 1 cup coconut milk 1 tablespoon butterscotch extract 1 cup Swerve 1/8 teaspoon xanthan gum 3 avocados, pitted, peeled and mashed

Directions

Place all ingredients in your blender. Process until well combined.Enjoy!

218. American-Style Mini Cheesecakes

(Ready in about 25 minutes | Servings 12) Per serving: 134 Calories; 12.5g Fat; 3.3g Carbs; 4.6g Protein; 0.4g Fiber

Ingredients

6 ounces Neufchatel cheese, at room temperature 7 tablespoons coconut oil, melted 5 eggs 1/4 teaspoon ground cinnamon 1/4 cup Swerve 2 ounces cocoa powder, unsweetened 1 teaspoon vanilla paste 1 teaspoon rum extract 1/3 teaspoon baking powder

Directions Beat the ingredients using your electric mixer on high speed. Line a mini muffin pan with 12 liners. Spoon the mixture into prepared muffins cups. Bake in the preheated oven at 350 degrees F for about 20 minutes.Bon appétit!

219. Peanut Butter Cupcakes

(Ready in about 10 minutes + chilling time | Servings 10) Per serving: 266 Calories; 28.1g Fat; 2.6g Carbs; 3.3g Protein; 0.5g Fiber

Ingredients

1 stick butter 4 tablespoons heavy cream 1 tablespoon Erythritol 1 cup peanut butter

Directions

Place a bowl over a saucepan of simmering water. Add in all of the above ingredients and stir continuously until well melted and blended. Spoon the batter into muffin cups lined with cupcake wrappers. Allow them to harden for about 1 hour in your freezer.Enjoy!

220. Old-Fashioned Walnut Candy

(Ready in about 1 hour | Servings 10) Per serving: 162 Calories; 14.6g Fat; 5.9g Carbs; 2.3g Protein; 1.7g Fiber

Ingredients

4 tablespoons walnuts, coarsely chopped 1 tablespoon rum 1/2 teaspoon pure vanilla extract 1/2 cup lightly toasted walnuts, chopped 1/2 cup chocolate, sugar-free 1/2 coconut oil, room temperature 4 ounces coconut cream 1/4 cup confectioners' Swerve

Directions

Melt the coconut oil in a double boiler and fold in the coconut cream and confectioners' Swerve; stir to combine well. Remove from the heat and add in the rum, vanilla extract and chopped walnuts. Let it cool to room temperature. Roll into 20 balls and chill for about 50 minutes. Then, melt the chocolate and dip each ball into the chocolate glaze. Roll your candies in the chopped walnuts until well coated.Bon appétit!

221. Cashew and Pecan Fat Bombs

(Ready in about 40 minutes | Servings 12) Per serving: 114 Calories; 10.6g Fat; 3.4g Carbs; 3.1g Protein; 1g Fiber

Ingredients

2/3 cup pecans, chopped 10 drops Monk fruit powder 1 teaspoon vanilla essence 1/4 cup almond flour 2 tablespoons cocoa powder, unsweetened 1/2 cup cashew butter 1/2 cup coconut oil

Directions

Mix all ingredients in a bowl until well combined. Drop by teaspoonfuls onto foil-lined baking sheets. Chill in your refrigerator until firm.Bon appétit!

222. Easy Coconut Mousse

(Ready in about 15 minutes+ chilling time | Servings 6) Per serving: 303 Calories; 30g Fat; 3.1g Carbs; 3.5g Protein; 2.7g Fiber

Ingredients

1/2 cup coconut milk A pinch of grated nutmeg 1 cup double cream 1/2 cup panela cheese 2 tablespoons powdered Erythritol 1/2 cup coconut creamer 1 ½ cups avocado, pitted, peeled and mashed

Directions

Warm the coconut milk and creamer over low heat. Remove from the heat. Stir in the avocado and nutmeg; continue to stir until everything is well incorporated. Add in the remaining ingredients. Beat using an electric mixer on medium-high speed. Place in your refrigerator until firm.Enjoy!

223. Cheesecake Squares with Berry Topping

(Ready in about 30 minutes | Servings 6) Per serving: 333 Calories; 28.4g Fat; 6.3g Carbs; 11.7g Protein; 0.1g Fiber

Ingredients

For the Cheesecake Squares:

1 cup soft cheese 1 teaspoon vanilla essence 3 tablespoons Swerve 1/2 cup butter, melted 4 eggs

For the Berry Topping:

1/2 teaspoon lime juice 1 ½ tablespoons coconut milk 3/4 cup, frozen mixed berries 2 tablespoons Swerve

Directions

Start by preheating your oven to 340 degrees F. Line a baking pan with a Silpat mat. In a mixing bowl, combine all ingredients for the cheesecake squares using an electric mixer. Press the crust into the baking pan. Bake in the preheated oven for about 23 minutes. Warm all of the topping ingredients in a saucepan over a moderate flame. Reduce the heat to a simmer and continue to cook until the sauce has reduced by half. Spoon the berry topping over the chilled cheesecake.Bon appétit!

224. Greek-Style Coconut Cheesecake

(Ready in about 30 minutes | Servings 12) Per serving: 246 Calories; 22.2g Fat; 5.7g Carbs; 8.1g Protein; 1.9g Fiber

Ingredients

5 ounces Greek-style yogurt 1 ounce coconut flakes 10 ounces almond meal 1/4 teaspoon grated nutmeg 1 teaspoon lemon zest 5 ounces soft cheese 1 teaspoon baking powder 4 eggs, lightly beaten 4 ounces Swerve 1/4 coconut oil

Directions Brush two spring form pans with a nonstick spray. Mix the almond meal, coconut flakes, nutmeg, and baking powder. Add in the eggs, one at a time, whisking constantly; add in 2 ounces of Swerve. Spoon the mixture into spring form pans and bake at 360 degrees F for 23 minutes. In another bowl, combine the coconut oil, lemon zest, yogurt, soft cheese, and the remaining 2 ounces of Swerve. Mix to combine and spoon the filling over the first crust. Spread half of the filling over it. Top with another crust and spread the rest of the filling over the top.Bon appétit!

225. **The Best Keto Birthday Cake**

(Ready in about 40 minutes + chilling time | Servings 10) Per serving: 241 Calories; 22.6g Fat; 4.2g Carbs; 6.6g Protein; 0.7g Fiber

Ingredients

For the Cake Base: 2/3 cup coconut flour 2 ½ tablespoons butter 4 eggs 1 cup full-fat milk 1 teaspoon vanilla extract 1 ½ cups almond meal 1/2 teaspoon baking powder A pinch of coarse salt 1 cup erythritol

For the Frosting: 1/3 cup erythritol 3 ounces coconut oil, at room temperature A few drops coconut flavor 10 ounces soft cheese

Directions

Mix all ingredients for the cake base until well combined. Press the crust into a parchment-lined springform pan. Bake at 365 degrees F for 30 minutes or until a toothpick comes out clean; allow it to cool to room temperature. Meanwhile, beat the cheese using your electric mixer until creamy. Stir in the remaining ingredients and continue to mix until well combined. Frost your cake and serve well-chilled.Bon appétit!

226. **Decadent Macchiato Penuche**

(Ready in about 10 minutes + chilling time | Servings 8) Per serving: 145 Calories; 12.8g Fat; 6.2g Carbs; 0.9g Protein; 1.2g Fiber

Ingredients

1 teaspoon warm coffee 1 teaspoon caramel flavor 6 tablespoons butter 1 tablespoon peanut butter 3 ounces dark chocolate, unsweetened 1 teaspoon liquid Monk fruit

Directions

Microwave the butter and chocolate until they are completely melted. Fold in the remaining ingredients. Spoon the batter into a foil-lined baking pan, smoothing out the top. Place in your refrigerator for 30 minutes before cutting. Enjoy!

227. **Coconut and Peanut Bark**

(Ready in about 10 minutes + chilling time | Servings 12) Per serving: 316 Calories; 31.6g Fat; 4.6g Carbs; 6.6g Protein; 2.6g Fiber

Ingredients 3/4 cup coconut oil 1/2 teaspoon pure almond extract 1/2 cup coconut, shredded 3/4 cup peanut butter 1 cup powdered Erythritol

Directions

Melt all ingredients in a double boiler over medium-low heat. Scrape the batter into a parchment-lined baking pan. Place in your freezer for about 1 hour; break your bark into pieces.Bon appétit!

228.   Orange Crème Brûlée

(Ready in about 45 minutes + chilling time | Servings 5) Per serving: 205 Calories; 16.4g Fat; 6.5g Carbs; 7.4g Protein; 0g Fiber

Ingredients

3/4 cup Erythritol 6 eggs 1 ½ cups double cream 1 teaspoon orange rind, grated 1 teaspoon orange juice 1/2 teaspoon star anise, ground 3/4 cup water

Directions

In a saute pan, melt Erythritol until it has caramelized. Spoon the caramelized Erythritol into 5 ramekins. Bring the cream along with water to a boil. Whisk the eggs until pale and frothy; add in the remaining ingredients and stir to combine well. Add the mixture to the warm cream mixture and stir to combine well. Spoon the egg/cream mixture over the caramelized Erythritol. Lower the ramekins into a large cake pan. Pour hot water into the pan to come halfway up the sides of your ramekins. Bake at 325 degrees F for about 45 minutes. Refrigerate for at least 2 hours.Enjoy!

229.   Chocolate Marshmallows

Ready in about: 30 minutes | Serves: 4 Per serving: Kcal 55, Fat 2.2g, Net Carbs 5.1g, Protein 0.5g

Ingredients

2 tbsp unsweetened cocoa powder ½ tsp vanilla extract ½ cup swerve sugar 1 tbsp xanthan gum A pinch Salt 2 ½ tsp gelatin powder

Directions

Dusting 1 tbsp unsweetened cocoa powder 1 tbsp swerve confectioner's sugar Line the loaf pan with parchment paper and grease with cooking spray. Mix the xanthan gum with 1 tbsp water and pour it into a saucepan. Stir in the swerve sugar, 2 tbsp of water, and salt. Place the pan over medium heat and bring the mixture to a boil. Reduce the heat and simmer for 7 minutes. Cover the gelatin with cold water in a small bowl. Let sit there without stirring to dissolve for 5 minutes. While the gelatin dissolves, pour the remaining water into a small bowl and heat in the microwave for 30 seconds. Stir in cocoa powder and mix it into the gelatin. When the sugar solution has hit the right temperature, gradually pour it directly into the gelatin mixture while continuously whisking. Beat for 10 minutes to get a light and fluffy consistency. Next, stir in the vanilla and pour the blend into the loaf pan. Let the marshmallows set for 3 hours and then use an oiled knife to cut them it into cubes; place them on a plate. Mix the remaining cocoa powder and confectioner's sugar together. Sift it over the marshmallows.

230. Coconut Cheesecake

Ready in about: 30 minutes + freezing time | Serves: 12 Per serving: Kcal 256, Fat: 25g, Net Carbs: 3g, Protein: 5g

Ingredients

Crust 2 egg whites ¼ cup erythritol 3 cups desiccated coconut 1 tsp coconut oil ¼ cup melted butter Filling 3 tbsp lemon juice 6 oz raspberries 2 cups erythritol 1 cup whipped cream Zest of 1 lemon 24 oz cream cheese

Directions

Grease the bottom and sides of a cake pan with coconut oil. Line with parchment paper. Preheat oven to 350°F and mix all crust ingredients. Pour the crust into the pan. Bake for about 25 minutes; let cool. Meanwhile, beat the cream cheese with an electric mixer until soft. Add the lemon juice, zest, and erythritol. Fold the whipped cream into the cheese cream mixture. Fold in the raspberries gently. Spoon the filling into the baked and cooled crust. Place in the fridge for 4 hours.

231. Berry Tart

Ready in about: 45 minutes | Serves: 4 Per serving: Kcal 305, Fat: 26.5g, Net Carbs: 4.9g, Protein: 15g

Ingredients

4 eggs 2 tsp coconut oil 2 cups berries 1 cup coconut milk 1 cup almond flour ¼ cup sweetener ½ tsp vanilla powder 1 tbsp powdered sweetener A pinch of salt Preheat oven to 350°F.

Directions

Place all ingredients except coconut oil, berries, and powdered sweetener, in a blender; blend until smooth. Gently fold in the berries. Grease a baking dish with the oil. Pour the mixture into the prepared pan and bake for 35 minutes. Sprinkle with powdered sugar to serve.

232.   Passion Fruit Cheesecake Slices

Ready in about: 15 minutes + cooling time | Serves: 6 Per serving: Kcal 287, Fat 18g, Net Carbs 6.1g, Protein 4.4g

Ingredients

1 cup crushed almond biscuits ½ cup melted butter Filling 1 ½ cups cream cheese ¾ cup swerve sugar 1 ½ whipping cream 1 tsp vanilla bean paste 4-6 tbsp cold water 1 tbsp gelatin powder Passionfruit jelly 1 cup passion fruit pulp ¼ cup swerve confectioner's sugar 1 tsp gelatin powder ¼ cup water, room temperature

Directions

Mix the crushed biscuits and butter in a bowl, spoon into a spring-form pan, and use the back of the spoon to level at the bottom. Set aside in the fridge. Put the cream cheese, swerve sugar, and vanilla paste into a bowl, and use the hand mixer to whisk until smooth; set aside. Cover the gelatin with cold water in small bowl. Let dissolve for 5 minutes. Pour the gelatin liquid along with the whipping cream in the cheese mixture and fold gently. Remove the spring-form pan from the refrigerator and pour over the mixture. Return to the fridge. For the passionfruit jelly: add 2 tbsp of cold water and sprinkle 1 tsp of gelatin powder. Let dissolve for 5 minutes. Pour confectioner's sugar and ¼ cup of water into it. Mix and stir in passion fruit pulp. Remove the cake again and pour the jelly over it. Swirl the pan to make the jelly level up. Place the pan back into the fridge to cool for 2 hours. When completely set, remove, and unlock the spring-pan. Lift the pan from the cake and slice the dessert.

233.   Granny Smith Apple Tart

Ready in about: 65 minutes | Serves: 6 Per serving: Kcal 302, Fat: 26g, Net Carbs: 6.7g, Protein: 7g

Ingredients

6 tbsp butter 2 cups almond flour 1 tsp cinnamon ⅓ cup sweetener Filling 2 cups sliced Granny Smith ¼ cup butter ¼ cup sweetener ½ tsp cinnamon ½ tsp lemon juice Topping ¼ tsp cinnamon 2 tbsp sweetener

Directions

Preheat oven to 370°F and combine all crust ingredients in a bowl. Press this mixture into the bottom of a greased pan. Bake for 5 minutes. Remove and let it cool slightly. Combine the apples and lemon juice in a bowl and arrange them on top of the cooled crust. Combine the rest of the filling ingredients and brush the mixture over the apples. Bake for about 30 minutes. Press the apples down with a spatula, return to oven, and bake for 20 more minutes. Combine the cinnamon and sweetener in a bowl and sprinkle over the tart. Note: Granny Smith apples have just 9.5g of net carbs per 100g. Still high for you? Substitute with Chayote squash, which has the same texture and rich nutrients, and just around 4g of net carbs.

234. Chocolate Chip Cookies

Ready in about: 20 minutes | Serves: 4 Per serving: Kcal 317, Fat 27g, Net Carbs 8.9g, Protein 6.3g

Ingredients

1 cup butter, softened 2 cups swerve brown sugar 3 eggs 2 cups almond flour 2 cups unsweetened chocolate chips Preheat oven to 350°F.

DirectionsLine a baking sheet with parchment paper. Whisk the butter and sugar with a hand mixer for 3 minutes or until light and fluffy. Add the eggs one at a time, and scrape the sides as you whisk. Mix in almond flour at low speed until well combined. Fold in the chocolate chips. Scoop 3 tablespoons each on the baking sheet, creating spaces between each mound, and bake for 15 minutes to swell and harden. Remove, cool, and serve.

235. Lemon Cheesecake Mousse

Ready in about: 5 minutes + cooling time | Serves: 4 Per serving: Kcal 223, Fat 18g, Net Carbs 3g, Protein 12g

Ingredients

24 oz cream cheese, softened 2 cups swerve confectioner's sugar 2 lemons, juiced and zested ¼ tsp salt 1 ¼ cups whipped cream

Directions

Whip the cream cheese in a bowl with a hand mixer until light and fluffy. Mix in the swerve sugar, lemon juice, and salt. Fold in 1 cup of the whipped cream to evenly combine. Spoon the mousse into serving cups and refrigerate to thicken for 1 hour. Swirl with the remaining whipped cream and garnish lightly with lemon zest. Let sit in the fridge before serving.

236. Chia & Blackberry Pudding

Ready in about: 10 minutes + chilling time | Serves: 2 Per serving: Kcal 169, Fat: 10g, Net Carbs: 4.7g, Protein: 7.5g

Ingredients

1 cup full-fat natural yogurt 2 tsp swerve sugar 2 tbsp chia seeds 1 cup fresh blackberries 1 tbsp lemon zest Mint leaves, to serve

Directions

In a bowl, mix the yogurt and swerve sugar. Stir in the chia seeds. Reserve 4 blackberries for garnish. Mash the remaining ones with a fork. Stir in the yogurt mixture. Put in the fridge for 30 minutes. Divide the mixture between 2 glasses. Top each with a couple of blackberries, mint, and lemon zest. Serve.

237.   Vanilla Chocolate Mousse

Ready in about: 30 minutes | Serves: 4 Per serving: Kcal 370, Fat: 25g, Net Carbs: 3.7g, Protein: 7.6g

Ingredients

3 eggs 1 cup dark chocolate chips 1 cup heavy cream 1 cup fresh strawberries, sliced 1 vanilla extract 1 tbsp swerve sugar

DirectionsMelt the chocolate in a bowl, in your microwave for a minute on high, and let it cool for 10 minutes. Meanwhile, in a medium-sized mixing bowl, whip the cream until very soft. Add the eggs, vanilla extract, and swerve; whisk to combine. Fold in the cooled chocolate. Divide the mousse between four glasses, top with the strawberry slices, and chill in the fridge for at least 30 minutes before serving.

238.   Blueberry Ice Pops

Ready in about: 5 minutes + cooling time | Serves: 6 Per serving: Kcal 48, Fat 1.2g, Net Carbs 7.9g, Protein 2.3g

Ingredients

3 cups blueberries ½ tbsp lemon juice ¼ cup swerve sugar Pour the blueberries, lemon juice, swerve sugar, and ¼ cup water in a blender, and puree on high speed for 2 minutes until smooth.

Directions

Strain through a sieve into a bowl, discard the solids. Mix in more water if too thick. Divide the mixture into ice pop molds, insert stick cover, and freeze for 4 hours to 1 week. When ready to serve, dip in warm water and remove the pops.

239.   Blackcurrant Iced Tea

Ready in about: 10 minutes | Serves: 4 Per serving: Kcal 22, Fat 0g, Net Carbs 5g, Protein 0g

Ingredients

½ cup sugar-free blackcurrant extract 6 unflavored tea bags Swerve to taste

Directions

Ice cubes for serving Lemon slices to garnish Pour the ice cubes in a pitcher and place it in the fridge. Bring 2 cups of water to boil in a saucepan over medium heat for 3 minutes and turn the heat off. Stir in the sugar to dissolve and steep the tea bags in the water for 2 minutes. Remove the bags after and let the tea cool down. Stir in the blackcurrant extract until well incorporated, remove the pitcher from the fridge, and pour the mixture over the ice cubes. Let sit for 3 minutes to cool and after, pour the mixture into tall glasses. Add some more ice cubes, place the lemon slices on the rim of the glasses, and serve the tea cold.

240. Almond Butter Fat Bombs

Ready in about: 3 minutes + cooling time | Serves: 4 Per serving: Kcal 193, Fat 18.3g, Net Carbs 2g, Protein 4g

Ingredients

½ cup almond butter ½ cup coconut oil 4 tbsp unsweetened cocoa powder ½ cup erythritol

Directions

Melt butter and coconut oil in the microwave for 45 seconds, stirring twice until properly melted and mixed. Mix in cocoa powder and erythritol until thoroughly combined. Pour into muffin molds and refrigerate for 3 hours to harden.

241. Berry Merry

Ready in about: 6 minutes | Serves: 4 Per serving: Kcal 83, Fat 3g, Net Carbs 8g, Protein 2.7g

Ingredients

1 cup strawberries + extra for garnishing 1 ½ cups blackberries 1 cup blueberries 2 small beets, peeled and chopped 2/3 cup ice cubes 1 lime, juiced

Directions

For the extra strawberries for garnishing, make a single deep cut on their sides; set aside. Add the blackberries, strawberries, blueberries, beet, and ice cubes into the smoothie maker. Blend the ingredients at high speed until smooth and frothy, for about 60 seconds. Add the lime juice, and puree further for 30 seconds. Pour the drink into tall smoothie glasses, fix the reserved strawberries on each glass rim, stick a straw in, and serve the drink immediately.

242.   Peanut Butter Pecan Ice Cream

Ready in about: 36 minutes + chilling time | Serves: 4 Per serving: Kcal 302, Fat 32g, Net Carbs 2g, Protein 5g

Ingredients

½ cup swerve sweetener confectioners 2 cups heavy cream 1 tbsp erythritol ½ cup smooth peanut butter 1 tbsp olive oil 2 eggs yolks ½ cup pecans, chopped

Directions

Warm heavy cream with peanut butter, olive oil, and erythritol in a small pan over low heat without boiling for about 3 minutes. Remove from the heat. In a bowl, beat the egg yolks until creamy in color. Stir the eggs into the cream mixture. Continue stirring until a thick batter has formed, about 3 minutes. Pour the cream mixture into a bowl. Refrigerate for 30 minutes. Stir in sweetener confectioners. Pour the mixture into the ice cream machine and churn it according to the manufacturer's instructions. Stir in the pecans after and spoon the mixture into a loaf pan. Freeze for 2 hours before serving.

243.   Mixed Berry Trifle

Ready in about: 3 minutes + cooling time | Serves: 4 Per serving: Kcal 321, Fat 28.5g, Net Carbs 8.3g, Protein 9.8g

Ingredients

½ cup walnuts, toasted 1 avocado, chopped 1 cup mascarpone cheese, softened 1 cup fresh blueberries 1 cup fresh raspberries 1 cup fresh blackberries

Directions

In four dessert glasses, share half of the mascarpone, half of the berries (mixed), half of the walnuts, and half of the avocado, and repeat the layering process for a second time to finish the ingredients. Cover the glasses with plastic wrap and refrigerate for 45 minutes until quite firm

244.   Chocolate Bark with Almonds

Ready in about: 5 minutes + cooling time | Serves: 12 Per serving: Kcal 161, Fat: 15.3g, Net Carbs: 1.9g, Protein: 1.9g

Ingredients

½ cup toasted almonds, chopped ½ cup butter 10 drops stevia ¼ tsp salt ½ cup unsweetened coconut flakes 4 oz dark chocolate

DirectionsMelt together the butter and chocolate, in the microwave, for 90 seconds. Remove and stir in stevia. Line a cookie sheet with waxed paper and spread the chocolate evenly. Scatter the almonds on top, coconut flakes, and sprinkle with salt. Refrigerate for one hour.

245.   Coconut Fat Bombs

Ready in about: 2 minutes +cooling time | Serves: 4 Per serving: Kcal 214, Fat 19g, Net Carbs 2g, Protein 4g

Ingredients

2/3 cup coconut oil, melted 1 (14 oz) can coconut milk 18 drops stevia liquid 1 cup unsweetened coconut flakes

Directions

Mix the coconut oil with the milk and stevia to combine. Stir in the coconut flakes until well distributed. Pour into silicone muffin molds and freeze for 1 hour to harden.

246.   Chia Pudding with Coconut and Lemon

(Ready in about 1 hour | Servings 4) Per serving: 270 Calories; 24.7g Fat; 6.5g Carbs; 4.6g Protein; 4g Fiber

Ingredients

1/3 cup chia seeds 1/2 cup Greek-style yogurt 1/3 teaspoon vanilla extract 1/2 teaspoon ground cloves 1/4 teaspoon ground cinnamon 1/2 cup coconut milk 1 cup coconut cream 2 tablespoons Erythritol

Directions Place all ingredients in a glass jar and let it sit in your refrigerator for 1 hour.

247.   Peanut Butter Fudge Cake

(Ready in about 3 hours | Servings 8) Per serving: 180 Calories; 18.3g Fat; 4.5g Carbs; 1g Protein; 1.1g Fiber

Ingredients

3/4 cup peanut butter, sugar-free, preferably homemade 3 tablespoons cocoa nibs, unsweetened and melted 1/4 teaspoon baking powder 3 tablespoons coconut oil, at room temperature 1 teaspoon vanilla extract 1 stick butter 1/3 cup almond milk 1/3 cup Swerve A pinch of salt A pinch of grated nutmeg

Directions Melt the butter in your microwave. Stir in the milk, 1/4 cup of Swerve, salt, nutmeg, and baking powder. Spoon the batter into a parchment-lined baking dish. Refrigerate for about 3 hours or until set. Meanwhile, make the sauce by whisking the remaining ingredients until everything is well incorporated. Spoon the sauce over your fudge cake.Enjoy!

248. Mom's Coconut Tarts

(Ready in about 40 minutes + chilling time | Servings 4) Per serving: 304 Calories; 27.7g Fat; 6.6g Carbs; 11.6g Protein; 1.5g Fiber

Ingredients

1 cup coconut cream, unsweetened A pinch of nutmeg 1/4 teaspoon ground cinnamon 1/2 cup granulated Erythritol 1 teaspoon pure almond extract 4 eggs 1/2 cup almond butter A pinch of salt

Directions

Melt the coconut cream in a sauté pan over medium-low heat. Remove form heat. Mix the remaining ingredients until well combined. Now, gradually pour the egg mixture into the warm coconut cream, whisking to combine well. Spoon the mixture into small tart cases. Bake in the preheated oven at 350 degrees F for about 30 minutes until they are golden and firm.Bon appétit!

249. Bourbon Vanilla Cheesecake

(Ready in about 30 minutes + chilling time | Servings 10) Per serving: 211 Calories; 19g Fat; 4.4g Carbs; 7g Protein; 0.5g Fiber

Ingredients

For the Crust:

2 tablespoons walnuts, chopped 4 tablespoons peanut butter, room temperature 1 cup coconut flour

For the Filling:

1/2 teaspoon vanilla essence 2 tablespoons bourbon 1 teaspoon fresh ginger, grated 10 ounces cream cheese, room temperature 2 eggs 1/2 teaspoon Monk fruit sweetener

Directions

Mix all of the crust ingredients. Press the crust into a parchment-lined springform pan and bake at 330 degrees F for about 10 minutes. Place the springform pan in a deep baking tray filled with 2 inches of warm water to help create steam during baking. Make the cheesecake filling by mixing all the ingredients using an electric mixer. Spread the filling onto the crusts and bake an additional 20 minutes.Bon appétit!

250. Easy Lemon Panna Cotta

(Ready in about 10 minutes + chilling time | Servings 10) Per serving: 221 Calories; 21.5g Fat; 3.8g Carbs; 4.3g Protein; 0g Fiber

Ingredients

1 teaspoon lemon juice 1 teaspoon lemon rind, grated 1 teaspoon vanilla extract 1 ½ teaspoons gelatins powder, unsweetened 1/2 cup almond milk 1 cup double cream 1/4 cup erythritol

Directions

Place the gelatin and milk in a saucepan and let it sit for 2 minutes. Add in the other ingredients and stir to combine. Let it simmer for 3 to 4 minutes until the gelatin has dissolved completely. Pour the mixture into 4 ramekins and transfer to your refrigerator; cover and let it sit overnight or at least 6 hours. Enjoy!

251. Frozen Walnut Dessert

(Ready in about 10 minutes + chilling time | Servings 6) Per serving: 84 Calories; 8.9g Fat; 1.5g Carbs; 0.8g Protein; 0.7g Fiber

Ingredients

1/2 stick butter, melted 1/2 teaspoon almond extract A few drops Monk fruit powder 2 tablespoons cocoa powder 2 tablespoons walnuts, chopped

Directions

Melt the butter in your microwave; add in the almond extract, Monk fruit powder, and cocoa powder. Spoon the mixture into a parchment-lined baking tray. Scatter the chopped walnuts on top and place in your freezer until set.Bon appétit!

252. Coconut and Berry Ice Cream

(Ready in about 10 minutes + chilling time | Servings 4) Per serving: 305 Calories; 18.3g Fat; 4.5g Carbs; 1g Protein; 2.7g Fiber

Ingredients

1 ¼ cups coconut milk 1/2 teaspoon xanthan gum 1/3 cup double cream A few drops Monk fruit 1/2 cup coconut flakes

Directions

In a mixing bowl, combine coconut milk, double cream, Monk fruit, and coconut flakes. Add in the xanthan gum, whisking constantly, until the mixture has thickened. Then, prepare your ice cream in the ice cream maker according to manufacturer's instructions.Bon appétit!

253.   Mixed Berry Scones

(Ready in about 25 minutes | Servings 10) Per serving: 245 Calories; 21.6g Fat; 7.4g Carbs; 3.8g Protein; 0.6g Fiber

Ingredients

1 cup mixed berries 1 ½ sticks butter 1 cup double cream 1 cup Swerve A pinch of salt A pinch of grated nutmeg 1 cup almond meal 1 cup coconut flour 1 teaspoon baking powder 2 eggs 1 teaspoon vanilla paste

Directions

Thoroughly combine the almond meal, coconut flour, baking powder, salt, nutmeg, and berries. In another bowl, whisk the eggs with the butter and double cream. Stir in Swerve and vanilla paste; stir until everything is well combined. Add the egg mixture to the almond flour mixture; stir until a soft dough forms. Shape the dough into 16 triangles and place them on a foil-lined baking sheet. Bake in the preheated oven at 360 degrees F for about 20 minutes.

254.   Greek Frappé Coffee

(Ready in about 2 hours | Servings 2) Per serving: 222 Calories; 15.8g Fat; 7.1g Carbs; 5.9g Protein; 0.3g Fiber

Ingredients

1 tablespoon cacao butter 1 cup almond milk 1/2 cup prepared instant espresso, cooled 1/2 teaspoon Monk fruit powder 2 tablespoons coconut whipped cream

Directions

In your blender, mix the cacao butter, almond milk, instant espresso, and Monk fruit powder until well combined.Enjoy!

255.   Old-Fashioned Walnut Cheesecake

(Ready in about 1 hour | Servings 14) Per serving: 393 Calories; 38g Fat; 4.1g Carbs; 9.8g Protein; 1.1g Fiber

Ingredients

The Crust: 1/3 cup Swerve 1/4 teaspoon ground cinnamon 8 ounces walnuts, chopped A pinch of salt 1 stick butter, melted 1/4 teaspoon ground cloves

For the Filling:

1 cup Swerve 1 teaspoon pure vanilla extract 4 eggs 14 ounces Greek-style yogurt 22 ounces Neufchâtel cheese, at room temperature

Directions

Mix all ingredients for the crust; press the mixture into a baking pan and set it aside Whip the Neufchâtel cheese using your electric mixer on low speed. Add in 1 cup of Swerve and vanilla. Fold in the eggs, one at a time, mixing constantly on low speed. Add in Greek-style yogurt and gently stir to combine. Bake in the preheated oven at 290 degrees F for 50 to 55 minutes. Bon appétit!

256.   Chocolate Nut Clusters

(Ready in about 15 minutes + chilling time | Servings 8) Per serving: 166 Calories; 17.2g Fat; 2.2g Carbs; 1.2g Protein; 1.1g Fiber

Ingredients

1/2 cup walnuts, chopped 1/2 cup coconut oil, at room temperature 1/4 cup cocoa powder, unsweetened 1/4 cup Erythritol A pinch of coarse salt

Directions

Melt the coconut oil in your microwave; add in cocoa powder and Erythritol. Remove from the heat and stir well. Add in the ground walnuts and coarse salt and stir until everything is well combined.   Drop by teaspoonfuls onto foil-lined baking sheets. Chill in your refrigerator until firm.Bon appétit!

257. Hazelnut Cake Squares

(Ready in about 30 minutes | Servings 8) Per serving: 241 Calories; 23.6g Fat; 3.7g Carbs; 5.2g Protein; 1g Fiber

Ingredients

2 cups almond meal 3 eggs 1 teaspoon almond extract 3/4 cup heavy cream A pinch of sea salt 1/2 cup coconut oil, at room temperature 1/2 cup hazelnuts, chopped 3/4 teaspoon baking powder 1 cup Erythritol 1/2 teaspoon ground cinnamon 1/4 teaspoon ground cardamom

Directions

Start by preheating your oven to 365 degrees F. Coat the bottom of your baking pan with parchment paper. Thoroughly combine the almond meal, baking powder, Erythritol, cinnamon, cardamom, and salt. After that, stir in the coconut oil, eggs, almond extract, and heavy cream; whisk until everything is well incorporated. Stir in the chopped hazelnuts. Scrape the batter into the prepared baking pan. Bake in the preheated oven for about 25 minutes.Enjoy!

258. Chocolate Jaffa Custard

(Ready in about 15 minutes | Servings 4) Per serving: 154 Calories; 13g Fat; 6.3g Carbs; 5.3g Protein; 1.7g Fiber

Ingredients

3 ounces cream cheese, at room temperature 2 egg yolks 1/4 teaspoon ground cardamom 1/4 teaspoon grated nutmeg 1/4 cup Swerve 1/4 cup cocoa powder, unsweetened 3/4 cup double cream 1 tablespoon orange juice, freshly squeezed

Directions

Whip the egg yolks using an electric mixer until pale and frothy. Warm the cream and gradually fold in the hot cream into the beaten eggs. Let it simmer for about 4 minutes, stirring continuously, until the mixture has reduced and thickened slightly. In another mixing bowl, beat the remaining ingredients until everything is creamy and uniform. Fold the avocado mixture into the egg/cream mixture; gently stir until well combined.Enjoy!

259.   Perfect Lemon Curd

(Ready in about 10 minutes + chilling time | Servings 6) Per serving: 180 Calories; 17.6g Fat; 5.2g Carbs; 2.8g Protein; 0.1g Fiber

Ingredients

4 ounces fresh lemon juice 1 ½ cups Erythritol A pinch of salt A pinch of nutmeg 2 eggs + 1 egg yolk, well whisked 1/2 cup butter, at room temperature

Directions

In a sauté pan, beat the eggs over a low heat. Add in the remaining ingredients and cook for about 5 minutes, whisking constantly. Turn the heat to the lowest setting and continue to stir with a wire whisk for 1 to 2 minutes longer. Cover with a plastic wrap.Enjoy!

260.   Autumn Pear Crumble

(Ready in about 30 minutes | Servings 8) Per serving: 152 Calories; 11.8g Fat; 6.2g Carbs; 2.5g Protein; 1.7g Fiber

Ingredients

2 ½ cups pears, cored and sliced 1/2 cup coconut flour 3/4 cup granulated Swerve 2 eggs, whisked 1/2 tablespoon fresh lime juice 1/3 teaspoon xanthan gum 3/4 cup almond meal 5 tablespoons butter

Directions

Preheat your oven to 365 degrees F. Brush the sides and bottom of a baking dish with a nonstick spray. Arrange your pears on the bottom of the baking dish. Drizzle the lime juice and xanthan gum over them. In a mixing dish, thoroughly combine the almond meal, coconut flour, and Swerve. Fold in the eggs, one at a time, mixing constantly until your mixture resembles coarse meal. Spread this mixture over the pear layer. Cut in the cold butter and bake in the preheated oven for 20 to 23 minutes or until golden brown on the top.Bon appétit!

CPSIA information can be obtained
at www.ICGtesting.com
Printed in the USA
BVHW091431070621
608934BV00003B/905